A LIFE WORTH LIVING:

Acting, Activism and Everything Else

A LIFE WORTH LIVING:

Acting, Activism & Everything Else

Tommy Jessop

WILDFIRE

First published in 2023 by
WILDFIRE
an imprint of HEADLINE PUBLISHING GROUP

1

Cataloguing in Publication Data is available from the British Library

Hardback ISBN 978 1 0354 0370 7

Typeset in Futura and Caudex by CC Book Production

Printed and bound in Great Britain by Clays Ltd, Elcograf S.p.A.

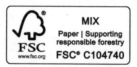

Headline's policy is to use papers that are natural, renewable and
recyclable products and made from wood grown in well-managed forests
and other controlled sources. The logging and manufacturing processes
are expected to conform to the environmental regulations
of the country of origin.

HEADLINE PUBLISHING GROUP
an Hachette UK Company
Carmelite House
50 Victoria Embankment
London EC4Y 0DZ

www.headline.co.uk
www.hachette.co.uk

To my fans and my loving family and to everyone who believes and supports me in everyday life.

To everyone living with Down syndrome, your extra chromosome makes you extra good company. I enjoy hearing about you all and what you are up to.

Always try to look on the bright side of life.

Contents

Preface

I have written this book because I'm a man on a mission to show that life with Down syndrome can be exciting and is worth living. I want other people to understand, and to give us the chance to live life to the full and to be fulfilled.

We are all different, with different gifts and skills. I'm a professional actor, dancer, campaigner and public speaker trying to make a difference, and I'm a Doctor of the Arts and now a writer. I'm also a brother, son, uncle, friend and best man. That is my story. Other people have their own exciting stories to tell.

After I was in the BBC TV series *Line of Duty* someone kindly offered to write a book about my life, but I

decided I wanted to write it myself, so here you are.
I really do hope you will enjoy yourselves reading my
memoir, and that it will not be too emotional for you –
or at least that it will be emotional for you in a good
way.

I will take you to award ceremonies, onto film sets
and behind the scenes, into my campaigns and
public speaking, tease you about sport and share
some emotional moments along the way. I will talk
about what it takes to play a character on stage or
on screen, and there might be a few puns. I quite
like puns! We might also talk about music and
Shakespeare and growing up.

There are some things I can't tell you about because
they have not come out yet and they are still top-
secret. I do find it difficult not being able to tell you,
but keeping secrets is all part of the life of an actor.

In some of my work there have been hard-hitting
stories, but these stories need to be told.

I hope this book can influence other people's lives,
and show how others have influenced my life as well.

Chapter 1

Truly alive

Being on stage really does make me come alive. Being on stage at the National Television Awards at the O2 Arena in London is something I will never forget. It was September 2021 and I was up there with the rest of the cast of *Line of Duty*, which had won two awards. The National Television Awards were celebrating the programme and they had invited me and other cast members, put us up in nice hotels in London and sent us cars to take us to the ceremony. I don't know what came over me, but suddenly I found myself dancing and doing a Brucie Pose in honour of Bruce Forsyth and it made the audience go wild. I felt so alive.

I also felt truly alive playing Hamlet. Standing on different stages in all sorts of venues and making the audiences feel Hamlet's deep emotions, even making them cry, is another thing I will never forget. There's something about Hamlet's situation and his speech 'To be, or not to be' that really connects with me and helps me express my emotions.

Standing on a famous stage in London, in the Sam Wanamaker Playhouse at the Globe Theatre in 2015, wearing my Hamlet costume and performing extracts from his speeches at a special event for Blue Apple Theatre made me feel even more alive.

I am writing this memoir to help people understand what my life is truly like. I really do want to change people's opinions and feelings about living with Down syndrome, and what it can be like when people give you chances in life. And to discover more about people with Down syndrome who are living their lives to the full.

I am really interested in finding out about other people, and I am a big fan of reading biographies and autobiographies. I have been inspired by so many people who have written books and memoirs that I thought I might try writing one about myself. It is quite intriguing and revealing to be writing my own story. It really does empower me and inspire me to find out what other people might be going through in their lives as well.

My life story has so far been quite wicked and brilliant. You will find out that 'wicked' really is my favourite word. I tend to use it mostly in a good way, when more positive things are happening in life. Some people use the word wicked to mean evil, but when I'm saying wicked I'm trying not to think about all the bad things in life. I think about the good things instead. To me wicked means it is all going well, but it is also a way of teasing people because it makes them laugh. If something bad is happening I don't really have a word for that. I mostly just go quiet. Wicked meant cool in the 1980s and 1990s when I was growing up and I love the word so much I have carried on using it.

One day I was reading the Bible in church. When I finished reading I said 'Wicked!' because I was happy. All the old ladies jumped. No one really expected me to say it, but I tend to get a kick out of using that word quite a lot. The word wicked in the Bible would mean evil, but on this occasion it meant I was pleased, a really good job done.

I might start off my story by describing myself as having two lives. One is just an ordinary happy life living with my family in a small city in England, hanging out with friends, volunteering at the local theatre and with a charity, and being a happy-go-lucky person who likes listening to music, quiz games, dancing and watching television programmes such as *Ant & Dec's Saturday Night Takeaway*, *The Voice UK* and *8 Out of 10 Cats* as well as *Who Wants to Be a Millionaire?* and *Beat the Chasers*. I like Nigella and Jamie Oliver's cooking shows and *Ready Steady Cook*, and checking out what's happening on *Strictly*. And not forgetting the football.

One thing you should know about me is that I am totally football-mad. I love doing a lot of research into all the transfer news. My killer question whenever I meet someone is asking them if they support a football team. It helps me understand them as a person, and sometimes we can have a laugh about things so it's a good icebreaker for me. I fancy myself as a bit of a football pundit, but don't worry if you don't like football: we can still be friends and talk about different interests, like films or other sports!

I support Newcastle United, because my brother William was born there. For a long time we have suffered as fans, but this season, while I have been writing this book, we are doing really well. Thank heavens for that! If we are lucky enough we could even end up winning something. It's been a very long time since Newcastle won a trophy. I really think it's our turn.

And my other life is being a professional actor, dancer, and activist who speaks in Parliament and tries to make things better for people with Down syndrome.

One of the most important moments in my career was playing Ben in *Coming Down the Mountain* for BBC One back in 2007. This was my first big professional acting break and it was nominated for a BAFTA

Award. I'm pretty sure that this was the first time I had ever seen anyone with Down syndrome on television, and it was myself I was watching. Others are playing Terry Boyle in *Line of Duty*, which has been watched around the world, playing Hamlet to over 2,000 people on different stages across the south of England, and becoming a full member of BAFTA. I will tell you more about these as we go along, but I think the moment that really changed my life was a pizza party. (We should have even more pizza parties, I reckon.) This was when I first told my mum and dad that I wanted to be a professional actor, but they did not actually listen. However, one person did listen to me, and thank heavens he did. I will tell you more about that in a bit.

Some people, like makeup artists, try to tease me by telling me that I look like Brad Pitt or Tom Cruise. It would be wicked to have a career like theirs. Maybe it is not mission impossible. (I did warn you that I enjoy making puns!) One person says I remind her of Hugh Grant. Well, I did have the same hairstyle as Hugh Grant when I met him, but he is a bit taller than I am. I have a wicked photo of us together at a launch event for Books Beyond Words and I still look at it with pride and joy. I enjoy the fact that I worked with Nicholas Hoult in my film *Coming Down the Mountain* and Hugh worked with Nicholas in his film *About a Boy*. Also, I do quite enjoy playing the villain, and Hugh had fun playing the villain in *Paddington 2*. I've played Henry F. Potter in *It's a Wonderful Life*, Marley's Ghost in *A Christmas Carol* and Frankenstein, which I really liked. Books Beyond Words is a great idea, by the way. They publish books that use pictures instead of words to help people with learning disabilities who are going through different things in life.

Lots of famous actors have been kind to me. Rory Kinnear's mum asked me if I would like him to send me a good luck card when I was playing Hamlet. I took her up on her offer and I still have the card. Russell Crowe sent me a 'well done' tweet for one of my short films. That was wicked.

It's not only actors who have been kind. Alan Shearer sent me a birthday card that I still treasure to this day. I think he is the best player Newcastle have ever had so far.

When I'm not working I just like to have fun and laugh, sing, dance and follow my football. Even though I have a very exciting life, the most important thing for me is my family and my friends. And what can I say about my very own mum?

Who knows what I would be doing if my mum had not founded Blue Apple Theatre and Low Level Circuits exercise group, and supported me in my professional career?

I really can give her praise for me coming in the world, and for being my mum. She is always there for me and I enjoy her company. I like making her laugh. I wondered what my mum would say about this, so I've asked her to tell me her memories of some things about my life that you might like to know as well. So, Mum, how about you fill in the gaps I can't remember, like when I was a baby, and what it has been like being with me in my career? I might be quite intrigued by what you have to say.

Tommy, your life so far has been completely extraordinary. From being told by a doctor that you would never learn to read, you have defied all predictions and eventually gone on to take on one of the most challenging roles in British theatre, and star in award-winning films and TV. I'm really looking forward to reliving some of these brilliant experiences we have shared together. I've had such fun with you. I never want our adventures to end!

I'm excited about writing this memoir. It really is about time people with Down syndrome should be able to speak up about what we would like to do and not just depend on other people saying things for us, but rely on ourselves. Other people can speak up about their choices in life; now it is time for people with Down syndrome to be able to do the same. I really am a man on a mission to show what living with Down syndrome is like. I want you to see that it is no different from being anyone else.

This is going to be just one man's story of a life worth living, and I hope people will enjoy reading it. One of my mottos in life is 'Don't judge a book by its cover.' So whether you are a person who has Down syndrome, or someone who has never even met anyone with Down syndrome, that is my message to you: don't judge a book by its cover. Except, of course, this one, which has an excellent cover. I really enjoyed the photoshoot with photographer Pål

Hansen. I had so much fun. I was having a joke with my brother William when that photo was taken. I was teasing him about which of us is the better-looking. Seeing the book jacket for the first time really did make me feel my life is worth living.

Chapter 2

Living with Down syndrome: don't judge a book by its cover

People living with Down syndrome are not all the same. We have different gifts and personalities, like any other group of people, and we can live and love and sing and dance and feel emotions like everyone else. I'm lucky because I've had great opportunities, but I believe that everyone has a gift; we just need to help them dig it out, then we will really see what they can do. We need to give people the chance to live life to the full. We need to tell our good stories so that other people are inspired to believe in us and help us follow our ambitions.

As a child I did not know that I had Down syndrome. I didn't find out until about twenty years later, when I got a lead role in a play about a boy who also had Down syndrome. I grew up feeling just like any other kid. Finding out didn't really make any difference to me because I understood that people with Down syndrome have something extra: an extra 21st chromosome. And that is a gift. It makes us special. One of the many perks of living with Down syndrome is that some of us are double-jointed, which might mean we are doubly special, actually. My party trick is to put both my feet behind my head.

I like to find out about the history of certain events, and one piece of my quite intriguing research is into the origin of the label 'Down syndrome'. Dr John Langdon Down first described our special features about 160 years ago, but I think we have always been around because archaeologists found the body of a child with Down syndrome who was carefully buried 5,500 years ago, having been breastfed by their mum. Then in the 1970s Dr Langdon Down's name started being used as a label for people like me.

That is just the label, though. I think this is a mixture of good and bad. The good thing is that I think that means people could and should understand us better. We should celebrate the lives of people living with Down syndrome. What is bad is being told what to do in life because of being labelled. This is why I have a personal grudge against labels. They separate us from making choices in life, because people just see a label and not the person. A label does not have a voice, but people with Down syndrome should start having their own voices heard. I myself might be a voice for those people who cannot speak up as such. So I might be a human version of a message being sent around the UK and the world. I really want to help improve other people's lives.

I have great sympathy for people who are not able to have their voices heard, and I really can relate to them because if anyone tells me what to do I do not react at all well. Beware of repercussions!

I don't really think about living with Down syndrome. I tend to just get on with my life. If I do think about Down syndrome it feels like a label, which is quite depressing. I might be different from others, but not because I have Down syndrome. I'm the exact opposite of many people, really. Other people tend to be serious, and I see the fun side of life and have a laugh.

I don't think Down syndrome is anything to be frightened of. It is part of me, but it is not who I am. I am a human being called Tommy Jessop, not a human being called Down syndrome.

I also have a grudge against labelling anyone with anything, really. I'm not sure it ever is helpful. I am a man on a mission to get rid all of the labels by seeing past them to what the person is truly like and what they are truly are capable of doing.

Chapter 3

Getting a kick out of life

Acting and dancing are two of the greatest passions in my life so far. On stage I've played all sort of roles over the years. I really love Shakespeare, and some of my favourite roles have been Hamlet, Prospero and Bottom. I enjoy making people laugh, like when I played the Mayor in Gogol's *Government Inspector* and Vladimir in Beckett's *Waiting for Godot*.

Apart from 'To be, or not to be', some of my favourite lines are 'We are such stuff as dreams are made of', 'People are bloody ignorant apes' (I'll explain that one later) and 'Why does everything smell of fish?'

One of my favourite acting experiences was performing Shakespeare to unsuspecting members of the public as part of the Cultural Olympiad in 2012. They generally did seem to be quite surprised, and it was really fun! I will tell you more about all this later on.

I've acted in films and TV shows, made documentaries and danced all over London, from Somerset House to art galleries and trendy stages in Hackney. Acting and dancing really make me come alive and let me show off my skills and talents, and what I truly am capable of.

Music has been a big influence in my life. Because I really am a human-being equivalent of music, I tend to be in a world of my own when I am listening to it. I actually like all kinds of music.

I also enjoy singing. Singing makes me feel more alive. I sound like Sir Tom Jones, apparently. The Welsh really are good singers, and I'm a quarter Welsh, which I am really proud of. I think that is how I have a really big voice, which I like using in the shower a bit too much.

Sometimes Dad and I play very loud music, such as Cat Stevens, the Rolling Stones, the Beatles, Cream or the Blind Boys of Alabama, and if Mum's there we all start dancing in the kitchen. But I also like ballads by Celine Dion, Adele and Whitney Houston, and Westlife's 'You Raise Me Up'. I danced to that for our dance-a-thons, which celebrate the lives of people with Down syndrome on World Down Syndrome Day. We used to dance for twenty-one hours on 21 March. This was inspired by the Church of England Synod voting 100 per cent for the motion 'We value the lives of people with Down syndrome.' That was the first time anyone had said anything like that to us. And S Club 7's 'Reach for the Stars' has to be one of my favourites. Mum says it's exactly what I am trying to do in my life.

I also have a stutter, which really is not helpful, but one way to get rid of it is by listening to rap music. And I like doing some beatboxing as well.

My idols in the world of music are Robbie Williams, Justin Timberlake, will.i.am and Little Mix. They are my guilty pleasure to listen to, by the way. And not forgetting Usher.

Recently I have begun to enjoy opera, including *Tosca* and *The Yeomen of the Guard*.

* * *

I also like researching things on the internet. These might include football transfer news, film reviews, music news and weather forecast updates. I enjoy looking up famous celebrities' birthdays and careers too, but I am also intrigued by facts about events happening in the world, in the past and the present. I might share a few intriguing facts as we go along. I like being quizmaster, and when I was little I used to take the box of Trivial Pursuit to my room and learn the questions and answers. I enjoyed doing that and surprising people when I knew the answers. Since then I've become a journalist in real life, finding out real facts – but more of that later.

I like the idea of being a pundit in life and sharing my opinions. I think the most important things for the world are peacemaking, climate change, food and safe homes. I do feel sorry for the homeless.

I am fascinated by what people think about how well their lives are doing. I can be an agony uncle, seeing what is going really well in other people's love lives and putting them on the right path to improve things if they seem to be going through a difficult patch. I can also be a bit of a mind reader and a comfort to other people if they are feeling sad or lonely at times. I like to know what people are thinking and whether they might be up to any mischief. I have to confess that I am a big fan of mischief. I love playing pranks on people, and I might even say that 1 April is one of my favourite days of the year.

Chapter 4

Casting can change the world

I've had fun playing all sorts of roles – from Shakespearean characters to a thief, a football fan, a fisherman and a boxer – but life as an actor is not always just about acting. There's lots of preparation before you film things or appear on stage, and there is quite a lot of work afterwards.

And you might be able to make a difference through film and TV work. For example, in *Holby City* I played a patient who wanted to make his own decision about an operation. His mum didn't want him to have it, so the story was all about who gets to decide and how to explain the situation so that the person involved, the patient with a learning disability, understands and can make their own choice.

In my short film *Fighter* I played a boxer who wanted to make his own decisions about his life, and whether to compete in boxing matches. I think this was based on a real-life person in America.

Not many bad things have happened to me personally, but in my work I have made training films and performed in plays for the NHS and the police about bad things that can happen so that people understand what is going on and can help. *Freddie's Story*, for example, which my brother Will and I made for Blue Apple Theatre, is a film about experiences in hospital with poor medical care and how to do things better, and *Living Without Fear* is a play about hate crime and mate crime.

Hate and mate crime can be problems for people who have learning disabilities, and often they don't know what to do about them. So we need TV and films to draw attention to them, and make sure people are more aware, notice things that are not right and help. This is part of my storyline in *Line of Duty* too.

Hate crime is when people are not very nice to you because of your disability or race or gender. Apparently Mencap found out that nine out of ten people with learning disabilities have been victims of hate crime, and that sadly this can happen over and over again. This means people are suffering over and over again, on a loop. This must stop right now.

Mate crime is when someone pretends to be your friend but maybe takes your money, or makes death threats, or bullies you to do things you don't want to do, leading you astray. Sometimes people might take over your home. This can also be known as cuckooing. I think it is important to say that it is not normal to be frightened of your friends or family. Small things can lead to much bigger things, like stealing money or dealing drugs, so you need to speak up and find someone you trust to help you get out of the situation. Please tell someone you trust straight away if this happens to you.

Tommy, your character in *Line of Duty*, Terry Boyle, was subject to cuckooing. This is an extremely distressing concept for anyone who cares for family members or friends who have Down syndrome and wants to support them to live as full and independent a life as possible. However, in order to enable them to live safely, we must be informed. So can you help us to understand this a bit more?

Cuckooing means you are stuck in a situation which you cannot get yourself out of, like having someone taking over your home and pretending to be your friend but in fact they are trying to get something out of you for money, or making you do something you don't want to. That might be anything from stealing your biscuits or your money to getting you caught up in dealing drugs, prostitution or any other crime.

In *Line of Duty*, Terry Boyle got framed for a murder which he did not actually commit. Bullies had taken over his flat and stored a dead body in his freezer. Viewers were shocked, but I think the story needed to be shown. Things like this really do happen, and they need to be prevented. Cuckooing is a matter of life and death in real life. So this is a powerful message to be sending out into the world. It is all about knowing how to make the right decisions, knowing when something is wrong, knowing how to speak up, and not giving in. Sometimes it is difficult to speak up, or you might be scared to do so, but you need to tell someone you trust if a bad thing happens. The trouble is, you need a voice to speak up and we need people to listen and check out our stories properly. Really listen to us. Don't think this cannot happen. Other people should also speak up for us or help us speak up if they notice anything that looks wrong.

As well as these roles in *Line of Duty* and *Living Without Fear* I've done other work that sends out an important message. In *Down and Out*, one of my short films, I had to play a victim when my on-screen brother got me shoplifting. In *Dead Fishes*, a BBC Radio 4 play with me and Hugo Speer, I played another victim whose brother got me accused of murder. Actually I have had quite a few evil older brothers on screen, which is funny, because in real life my older brother is not like that at all.

Living Without Fear came about a few years ago when the police asked Blue Apple to create a play about hate crime and mate crime. They wanted us to help them understand how to prevent people with learning disabilities from becoming victims. The script for *Living Without Fear* was written by my brother

Will, who did lots of research and spoke to lots of people about their experiences.

I played both a victim and a bully in the play. It certainly was quite something. I think it was important in getting across the message that we should be able to live without fear in our lives. We used dance as well as words to do this, and some people thought this helped them to understand it, and also to not be too upset by the stories we were telling. These were quite harsh and hard-hitting, especially when we read out newspaper reports of true stories of hate crime and of people being hurt and even killed in between the scenes we were acting.

We took a performance of *Living Without Fear* to Parliament at the invitation of Mr Speaker, who was John Bercow at the time. He asked us to perform it in his private apartment, and we invited ministers, MPs and Chief Constables from the police so that they could understand what it can be like having a learning disability and not knowing how to deal with bullying and mate crime or hate crime.

We had drinks beforehand and then performed our play. The performance went off really well and I think we sent out quite a powerful message. Some of the ministers, including Esther McVey, wanted to talk to us after the performance. Lord Alton, who was there, arranged for us take the play to schools around the country, and the Chief Constables invited us to perform it to police forces. They wanted to ask lots of questions too.

I remember you and the other actors talking to schoolchildren after one performance in the north of England. I was shocked, but not totally surprised, when a couple of sixth formers said they didn't realise that people with learning disabilities had feelings or could get upset if they were bullied. This is why it is so important to represent people with Down syndrome in our media. There is no substitute for meeting someone in person, but at least seeing you on screen should help viewers understand and value you all.

We found out then that some young people didn't realise we had feelings too. They didn't realise that it is upsetting for anyone to be called names. But we talked to them after the play and then everyone wanted to help.

I also would like to share what we learned when making *Living Without Fear* about how friends and family can help to keep people safe.

One of the best things is to encourage the person you care for to build safe friendship networks with other people who maybe also have a learning disability, or people from the wider local community, because loneliness can lead to relying on the wrong people. Perhaps there are activities they could join, like a local theatre group, a dance group or a sports club, so that they become known and recognised and have positive things they enjoy doing in their lives. In fact, the best support you can give someone is to be there for them and help them not to be lonely, because loneliness makes you vulnerable.

Where we live there is a 'Safe Places' scheme with certain local shops, supermarkets, coffee shops, a pizza restaurant and the local discovery centre. If someone is worried about anything they can go to these places and talk to someone.

Tell your person how much you love and value them, so that they realise their worth as a human being and are more confident. Maybe just try saying hello to someone on the street – as long as you don't put them on the spot or require them to respond. This can make a huge difference to someone's mood or self-esteem. A smile or kind greeting can mean a great deal. Don't be scared of feeling awkward.

We should not be victims at all. We do have our own ideas about life, our hopes and dreams.

My next ambition is to play a character who saves the day by making their presence felt. I did save the day in *Innocence*, one of my short films, although you might have to see what you think about the ending!

Now it is time for the TV and film industries to really listen to us and our life stories and give us positive roles. We can play characters who are truly like who we really are, or who are fantasy. These characters should also have a voice.

It is really important to represent people like us on screen so that viewers understand us better and see that we are capable. *Ralph & Katie* on BBC television has made a really great start on this. The couple played by Sarah Gordy and Leon Harrop get married and we see the ups and downs of everyday married life for them.

We shouldn't always play victims or people who are defined by having Down syndrome instead of simply being part of a great story and making a difference in that story. I truly believe people with Down syndrome can play any role you throw at them. How many of you would have believed that we could take on Shakespeare?

When you were growing up, you always said you just felt like any other kid. We never talked much about having Down syndrome or made a fuss about it. We just treated you like our other children. It will be wonderful if, now that people like you are seen so much more often on TV, the first thing viewers will think when they see you is 'Oh, there is that actor we saw in…' rather than 'Oh, what is it like to have Down syndrome?'

Let us surprise you. A doctor once said I would never learn to read, but I ended up playing Hamlet – and now I'm writing a book.

Chapter 5

Every small step is a miracle

My family is kind, supportive and loving. My dad is a retired doctor and my mum, who as I have said founded Blue Apple Theatre, is now my manager. I have an older brother who is a film director and a younger sister who is a filmmaker and writer.

No one expected me to do much when I was born. So how did I get from there to here? Come with me on a journey now and find out how this happened. I've also asked my mum to tell you more about when I was a baby because I can't remember much about that!

One dark, snowy January night in the north of England, baby Tommy decided to arrive a month early. This was just the first way in which he would surprise us. I started feeling the pangs of labour, but because it was too soon I leaned against a doorpost for a while and then continued putting our almost-two-year-old son William to bed. My husband was away so I wanted just to rest and wait, but something told me to pack my bag. I timed the pains and, just before midnight, phoned the hospital. The midwife wanted me to go in: I was definitely in labour. It was complicated, it was very late, and when I phoned the friends who had offered to look after William they didn't hear the phone ringing. Eventually someone did answer. It was my last resort: my husband's boss's wife who lived forty minutes away. When she arrived, I called an ambulance. We had a long, sloping drive and the snow made it impossible for the ambulance to reach the house. So I had to slither and slide down the snowy slope while in labour, leaning on the arm of the paramedic.

Tommy was born at 6 a.m. and I was left alone, shivering with cold and shock, in the middle of the gloomy delivery suite, by hospital staff who could not bear to tell me that he had Down syndrome. The only person I saw was a young midwife who walked past crying.

Those doctors and nurses never saw the toddler who became the smiliest, rosiest-cheeked little lad, who bounced up and down laughing with happiness whenever we walked into a room. Little did they know the fun and joy he would bring into our lives.

Little did I know then either, Tommy, of how you would travel the world and take us to wonderful places and events! It is true that as a baby you were not very well. It is also true that one doctor told me you would never read. Well that just shows how wrong doctors can be!

I went into a robotic mood and carried on. When people need to be looked after, you just do your best. As a tiny baby you took about eight hours a day to feed. My mother was staying to help, and I remember saying to her how amazing it was to discover I was fighting so hard to keep such a tiny and ill baby alive when, we thought, he might have so few prospects. But I was not fighting alone for you. Your dad and granny were there and someone from the next village shopped and cooked for us. But it was not just the kindness of family and the kindness of strangers. No, I believe God was fighting for you, our baby, too.

I didn't really know God then, but I surprised myself on the first day of your life when I learned that you had Down syndrome by suddenly asking 'Why has God sent this baby to us?' Then I thought, 'Oh, I believe in God.' Since then various friends who prayed for you when you were little said that they believed God had a purpose for you. I can still remember my lovely father holding you on his knees and hugging you very very tightly while he prayed for you. It was as if he was immersing you in love.

When you were almost a year old you were still not doing well, so much so that one of my friends was praying for you either to be healed or taken to heaven. You were healed. It was as if you slowly 'woke up' and became our wonderful loving, happy Tommy. Now people tweet and email thanking you for changing their lives through your work and campaigning. In some ways you have become a social engineer, an engineer of change for others who have Down syndrome.

We were lucky enough to be the first family in Cumbria to have the Portage home-visiting scheme. Named after the US town where it was invented, Portage is an educational system for children with learning disabilities which breaks down tasks into tiny steps. For example, if you are trying to teach a child how to dress themselves, you put most of their coat on but let them push their hand the last bit of the way down their sleeve. Gradually, day by day, they move towards putting on the whole sleeve themselves and eventually they manage the whole coat.

When the lovely woman from the Portage scheme arrived you were a very long way from dressing yourself. You were not even reacting to sounds. You were only a few months old, but, even so, she gave us ways to try to stimulate your awareness of your surroundings and your own senses. These included massaging across your body so that you would become aware of your feet and hands and later, when you were sitting up and crawling, playing with toys like balls or cars that could be pushed out of sight, encouraging you to crawl round the door to find them.

I might leave the rest of the babyhood stories to my mum to fill you in with the stuff that I cannot remember much about.

I was worried about leaving Tommy's older brother William out of all this lovely playtime, but our Portage friend made sure she played with him first for a while, before she turned to Tommy. When I was still having to feed Tommy for several hours a day, I used to tuck William under my other arm for a cuddle and read to him, or talk to him while he did jigsaw puzzles at my feet.

For several months, baby Tommy would hardly react to anything except the light sound of two bells on a stick or the gentle playing of nursery rhymes from a musical box. This love of music stayed with him. When he was about seven years old, his Saturday music club was really pleased because he had managed to read simple music and get the difference between a crotchet and a quaver when he was playing a tambourine. Growing up he loved singing and dancing – he still does, and he's certainly not the only one. We have lots of fun playing loud music and dancing crazily round the kitchen.

Music is one of my greatest passions in life. It makes me feel even more alive. It's quite rare that I get stressed out, but when I do I always listen to music. With some music I can't stop myself from dancing. I become the music itself and I seem to flow through it.

You woke up just after your first birthday. That is about the only way to describe it. You became the loveliest, smiliest toddler. It took you a while to toddle, but you would be sitting playing in your blue velvety dungarees with perhaps a stripy T-shirt, and when anyone came into the room you would bounce up and down, holding your hands forward and smiling the biggest, rosiest smile.

Tommy, you magnified the excitement of seeing a child learn because every small step was a miracle. Watching you develop almost in slow motion for the first few years made me want to understand how children learn and how their minds change. It's fascinating. Every parent would benefit from this knowledge, and from knowing that sometimes children are just not old enough to understand what we expect from them.

You always responded so well to praise and joy. It wasn't difficult to say well done and be excited about you learning new skills because you were so smiley. You were never naughty until you were about ten or twelve and then, funnily enough, we rejoiced! We rejoiced because it showed you were thinking for yourself!

I did nick someone's car keys once. I did that without people noticing. The person didn't realise their keys had gone. I hid them for a long while, then, when they did realise, I showed them I had the keys. I think when they knew it was me they saw the funny side and laughed. I warned you I do like being mischievous!

When I was little my sister and I used to share a double buggy, and then we started going to the village playgroup together. We used to sit on the floor looking at books together. I still enjoy her company. She is a very huggable, loving sister who is always supportive. She used to cuddle me when I was little and was crying. I always feel better when I see her, even now. She understands me and I love seeing her. She is a talented artist and writer. Once she drew my knees and Mum hung the picture on our wall – it is still there. Mum says she would always know those were my knees.

You first went to a playgroup in our village. Then, when you were about three, to Hillside, a special school in Sudbury, Suffolk, three days a week and the village school in Pebmarsh two days a week.

I think I quite enjoyed going to school. I went to six different schools, though I do not remember much about the first ones.

Do you remember the pancake race?

How could I not? It was at the village school when I was about six years old and when we flipped our pancake it landed on my head!

Apparently you were all running along with pancakes in little frying pans, trying to toss them. You were still all laughing about it when I collected you from school that day.

Hillside School was brilliant in many ways. You had a lovely teacher, Mrs Windley, who always told us what you could do and not what you could not do. She was as excited as we were about every tiny new thing you were managing to do or learn.

One strong memory is of walking out of school on your first day there. The headteacher followed us out and stopped me to talk. He asked how well you were eating and gave some very good advice. He pointed out that some people with Down syndrome have large tongues and find starting solid food quite annoying. He advised me to begin with something soft like banana and push the pieces back in if you pushed them out. Encouraging little children to chew properly like this is really important because it helps develop muscles for speaking clearly.

At that time you and your sister were both in highchairs and meals were fun, happy times.

My favourite food now is pizza, sausages, meatballs, pasta, steak, and pears, grapes, oranges, apples and strawberries. My favourite food when I was little was shepherd's pie or fish pie and Marmite sandwiches and bananas. Then I added in treacle tart and apple crumble and ice cream.

Babies with Down syndrome can have weak muscle tone, so exercises are important and can help later when they are learning to walk, do up buttons or start writing. I still do my exercises now because it is really important to get your daily dose of exercise and keep healthy, eating well and staying well.

It was heart-rending when we had to move away from Pebmarsh because Dad's job moved. You were very settled at schools where people seemed to love you. I will never forget finally closing the door and saying goodbye to our house, and then going to collect you from the village school. All fifty children rushed to the school gate crying out 'Why are you taking Tommy away, please don't take him away.' Tears ran down my face as we did up your seatbelt, started the engine and drove our little family out of the village.

It took time to find a new house, so for a term I taught you, William and your sister at home. We roosted in my parents' house and turned their dining room into a schoolroom. I discovered just how much you can learn when you teach in such small numbers. I was really teaching each of you one to one, leaving your brother to get on with, say, sums while I helped you with your writing.

Tommy, I still have your home schoolbooks from that time. When we started, you were beginning to trace over letters and numbers and form them yourself, understand simple counting sums and write the answers to simple comprehension questions. After a couple of months, you were writing short sentences using just three words and a picture to prompt you. We made a paper clock together and learned the time and you did a lot of colouring in to help with your fine-motor-control skills. I remember taking you all outside most days to see whether we could find any birds or insects or other wildlife, and to run around or kick a football and let off steam. Afterwards, we would lie on the floor listening to music like Tchaikovsky's rousing 1812 Overture, or the more gentle 'The Lark Ascending' by Ralph Vaughan Williams, and see whether the music helped us see stories or pictures in our heads.

When you were about eight years old, you suddenly learned to read. It seemed to happen overnight. One day you couldn't read. Next day you were reading.

Well at first I did find it quite difficult reading really long words, but that was a long time ago. I do

remember I found it quite easy reading. How could I not remember sitting with you or Dad reading the Biff, Chip and Kipper books? And I loved *Winnie the Pooh* and *The Wind in the Willows*, *The Famous Five* and *The Secret Seven* and *Just William*. Now I enjoy our night-time reading sessions and the books we've read like *The Explorer*, *The Ickabog* and *Jennings*, which is a laugh a minute and brings back happy memories of listening to tapes in the car.

When we moved house I went to a different local school in a new area. I went to two schools, the local school part-time and a special school, Shepherds Down, part-time. It was at Shepherds Down that I appeared in my first play as a snowman in a white fluffy costume.

At the local school, I helped some boys with their reading and they helped me with maths. My favourite books which helped me learn to read were the Biff, Chip and Kipper books. I remember one of the stories was about going to Buckingham Palace.

That reminds me of a real highlight in my childhood: meeting the Queen and Prince Philip. Recently the United Kingdom celebrated the Queen's life and four billion people watched on television, which is about half the world's population, apparently.

When I met Her Majesty the Queen, there were just the two of us in the back of her car. I was fortunate to have the chance to do this.

Here is how it happened. I was six years old and I was waiting with my mother to wave to the Queen as she was leaving the Bishop of Winchester's palace after lunch. Prince Philip noticed me standing there with my flowers. He beckoned me over and said 'Would you like to give your flowers to the Queen?' The Queen was already sitting in her car. Prince Philip gestured to me to go to the car to give the Queen her flowers, but I had to climb up a step and actually get into the car with Her Majesty to give them to her. My flowers got a bit squashed while I was climbing in. I was only little and the step was quite high for my short legs.

I think the Queen was a bit surprised to see me, a six-year-old boy, in her car when she was expecting Prince Philip to get in beside her. I was pleasantly surprised too to find myself there.

We had spent the morning waiting to see the Queen and looking at her big shiny car with a flag and no number plate. So I think it really was quite wicked just being in her car and meeting her.

At the Queen's funeral there were thousands of people marching in their uniforms, sailors, soldiers, airmen and women, heralds wearing red and gold, trumpets, cannons firing, bells ringing, bagpipes and bands playing, and the Royal Family walking behind her coffin.

When I met her it was really quiet – just me and her. Thank you, Prince Philip, for your kindness. It was an honour and something I will never forget.

A quick fact about the Royal Family:

The oil for anointing King Charles III at his coronation was made in Jerusalem from olives from the Mount of Olives. It has been perfumed with sesame, rose, jasmine, cinnamon and orange blossom. I wonder what it smelled like. They used to use ambergris from whales, but this time they did not use any animal products.

Chapter 6

'I want to be an actor'

People always ask how I started my career, which I do not mind talking about at all. I would like to let people know why I became an actor.

My first theatre work on stage was as that snowman at Shepherds Down when I was six. Around that time, though, I wanted to be a footballer. Then I literally changed my mind. I decided I wanted to be an actor when I was about ten. I just liked to make people feel happy and laugh.

When I was a teenager, I was a coaching assistant training up other boys at the Young Saints sessions at Henry Beaufort School. This was football for junior boys run by Southampton Football Club. I enjoyed myself there, running about, talking to the boys, fetching footballs, blowing the whistle, which was fun, handing out trophies and receiving them! I was working with Darren, who was one of the coaches at Young Saints. I liked it when the boys were happy and enjoying themselves on the field, having a good time. I'd also done some work in local libraries and in the MVC music store, sorting out CDs. But I didn't really get to do much more acting after the snowman even though I secretly wanted to.

When I was eighteen and about to leave college, Mum and I got lots of people together, like my teacher, my football coach, friends and family. We had pizza, and they asked me: what would you like to do next?

At that time it was a new idea that a person with a learning disability could and should make their own plans for their daily life and where they wanted to live. Generally, people like Tommy would have been simply placed by Social Services in day care and residential homes according to where they had spaces. It seems incredible to me now that as recently as 2003 we had to teach Tommy and people like him that they could make choices and own their own lives.

Tommy had invited everyone important to his life including Darren, his imaginative football coach, neighbours, smiley and warm and friendly as ever, church friends and members of his family; his father jovial, his sister calm and kind, his brother home from university and wondering what all this was about.

The only person missing was Martin Nobbs, a social worker. He was not Tommy's social worker – Tommy didn't have a social worker – but he knew Tommy from some football sessions he had been able to join. Although we didn't know it at the time, Martin was going to be key to all that has happened since.

In the middle of the table I had placed a large sheet of wallpaper on which I had written all the things Tommy had achieved and what we felt he was good at. We wanted to show him we had noticed he had done well and how proud of him we were. Then it would be up to him to tell us what he found easy, what he found hard and what he felt he was good at. He could tell us about his dreams and what he'd like to do next in his life. It was his chance to decide his own future, or at least the first steps towards his future.

How was he going to fill his week after leaving college? He was doing well supporting Darren as an assistant football coach, he loved reading, he was good at stacking CDs onto shelves in the right order in a music shop, he was kind, funny and had managed several work experience placements, including in a library, and seemed to enjoy it. We discussed working in the library and more football coaching responsibilities. One neighbour offered to take him swimming. But what was Tommy's dream?

He told us he wanted to be an actor.

I think that pizza party was the moment that actually changed my life. When I told them I wanted to be a professional actor Mum and Dad literally didn't believe me. I think they were probably in shock, but I felt it would be all right in the end. They had thought I might like to work in a library again. That had been fun, but I did think that being an actor might be even more fun. Well, I reckon I made the right decision.

This just shows how important it is to really listen to people: not just to let them speak, but to really hear what they are saying. At that moment, we failed as parents! We didn't take Tommy seriously. We felt that was what all young people at the time were saying. It seemed to me that everyone wanted to be on TV, so we rather dismissed Tommy's idea. So much for being person-centred!

Only Martin, who wasn't even sitting round this table because he thought we would be in a pizza place instead of at home, somehow heard about what I said and took note. He came round a few days later. He said he knew someone, and would I like to audition for a play. I might be truly thankful for small mercies and for Martin Nobbs!

I did not attend drama school. There wasn't one near enough that I could get to. But I did want to be an actor from a very young age. I reckon that people who are living with Down syndrome really should go into acting if that is their dream.

Because Martin listened, really listened, Tommy had the chance to audition for his first play. I was quite surprised when he suggested an audition, but this was the beginning of Tommy's acting career and he astonished us, setting the tone for the next few years! He continues to astonish us!

I did that audition, and I got the part. My first professional role was playing Adam in a play all about a person making choices in his life and being person-centred, instead of being told what to do and what not to do by other people. It was with the Phoenix Theatre in Bordon, Hampshire.

Ironically, the storyline was about a boy who wanted to be a chef, but his parents didn't listen!

I think that might have been the beginning of my campaigning, and standing up for anyone who is told they can't do stuff in life, when they really can. In the play, Adam wanted to make his own choice about getting a job. He was told he could not be a chef, but he proved everyone wrong. That is what I mean by looking past the label, seeing who people really are and helping them to dig out their gifts.

We took the play to schools and to the Chichester Festival Theatre.

This included a monologue and then a duologue in front of 600 schoolchildren on the massive Chichester Festival Theatre stage. I will never forget Tommy standing alone on that huge black apron stage as I watched from the wings, and how small he looked – a tiny brave figure in a vast expanse of blackness, with the golden spotlight on him. It was quite overwhelming.

The Phoenix Theatre Company then suggested that I could try taking part in the BBC/Channel 4 Talent Fund training for disabled actors. So in April 2004,

I went to an audition at the Oval Theatre in south London.

The journey to the audition was an adventure all on its own. We took the train to Waterloo and then the Underground, but as the Tube train pulled in I took a moment to double-check the Tube map.

Tommy climbed into the train and to my horror the doors began to close behind him. This was a serious moment. Tommy was very shy, new to London and likely to freeze if things went wrong. So I threw my bag between the doors and wedged them open. With considerable relief I managed to join Tommy, and we had a laugh, but I think we were both a little shaken.

How could I not remember this. The doors shut. I was on the train, you were on the platform. Not many things might have scarred me for life, but that was one of them.

At the Oval Theatre there were people from all over the south of England, with so many actors auditioning for the Talent Fund that there was an overspill into the Oval cricket ground.

They were also separately auditioning actors in the north of England. It just shows how many people had been waiting for this opportunity. Tommy was sent over the road with at least a hundred others to wait in the members' bar at the Oval cricket ground, and I remember being so tickled by being there that we phoned my father, who was a keen cricket fan.

I think the England cricket team were there. So the BBC/Channel 4 auditions were in one place and the England cricket team were in the other, which I thought was fun. I really wanted to go and see them at that point.

Finally Tommy was called in, but was back with me inside three minutes. I thought we could then leave, but someone came over and asked him to wait. After another long while he was called back in, and again was back out in just a few minutes. I never believed anything would come of this – there were so many people auditioning and many of them looked so confident. How would Tommy win a place, Tommy who had done so little acting so far?

For my audition I think I had a quick chat, but it was quite a long time ago – even before my first television role – so I can't remember much about it.

With this many people with all sorts of disabilities auditioning here and in the north and for you, Tommy, having so little acting experience, there were huge odds against you being accepted. But you gained a place on the scheme, one of only twenty-four actors, and one of only two who had learning disabilities.

I was quietly pleased when they said yes to me and I could go on the scheme. I was looking forward to all of it. I do not get nervous that much so it was just brilliant being accepted. I feel very grateful for the scheme. It was another of my personal highlights and I think it really started my career.

It was a wonderful programme of top-class training in London working with well-known directors, performance coaches, producers and casting directors in workshops and advice sessions. Tommy loved every minute and learned so much.

It was all to do with being well prepared in case TV and film roles came up in the future. We did some role-plays about how to get ready for auditions. There were role-plays where things went the right way and others when things went the wrong way, and we gave each other feedback on how well each person did and what they could improve on next time. I enjoyed taking part in all of it.

We learned about being in character and being in the moment, which means you are where the character is. We had to look into each other's eyes to see each other's reactions as well, which was really good fun.

There was lots of advice about looking for film and TV roles, and eventually it led on to *Coming Down the Mountain*, which was my first major TV role.

Then I was able to join Spotlight, which advertises actors and casting opportunities, and Equity, the actors' union. But it took time to get any more work.

We were later told that there was no writing for disabled actors, as commissioners and producers did not believe they would be able to find the talent to cast anyone until they had run the talent scheme and seen who they had available. Even ten years later, the feeling appeared to persist that there were not enough talented disabled actors to cast in meaningful roles. When roles did come up the storylines were often about problems associated with the character's learning disability, not about the lives they really led. As I write now there is a glimmer of hope, a breakthrough beginning to happen, as we start to see a few more people with Down syndrome in roles on television.

I just hope that by being in *Line of* Duty, *Coming Down the Mountain* and other TV and film shows I can help change people's minds so that they become more accepting of a diverse range of people.

Chapter 7

Taking the stage:
Blue Apple Theatre

I enjoyed the Talent Fund training and wanted to do more acting, but there were no roles on TV. So we looked for a theatre company instead, but at that time no one within reach would open their doors to me, an actor with Down syndrome. So there were no roles in theatre either.

There were only one or two theatre companies I could have joined. One place was the Chicken Shed in London, but it was a bit too far away. Mind the Gap was another one, but it was in Bradford and that was definitely too far away.

One day Mum had a phone call. 'Jane, have you seen the *Evening Standard*?'

It was our cousin Lisa. She is an actor and understood my need to perform, to be in character. She had read an article by Bill Nighy, who is one of my mum's favourite actors, about the Moment by Moment theatre group in London. That was also too far away, but Lisa asked 'Why don't you set up a theatre company yourselves?' That is how we came to set up Blue Apple Theatre.

That's right, Tommy! She gave us the inspiration to found a theatre company in our own area where you and others with learning disabilities could enjoy the stimulation and reward of appearing in live theatre. By setting it up ourselves, we could make sure there was no ceiling on our expectations of you all.

It took about six months to get going. First I had to persuade myself that it didn't matter that I had no experience as an actor or producer, because we could find someone to direct rehearsals. We just had to set things up. (That was me being naive.) The next thing was finding a venue, John Tellett at the Tower Arts Centre understood the vision and welcomed us there. To underscore the need, we ran a couple of pilot sessions in Summer 2005. They showed huge demand for a theatre group. Over fifty people turned up to each workshop and they all wanted to come back. They told me they were bored and lonely and had nothing to do.

Then we had to decide on a name which would make people want to know more, find a drama leader and, of course, get hold of some funding. We thought the name Blue Apple Theatre would be memorable and it certainly does prompt people to ask questions. So it works!

Blue Apple provides a theatre 'family' where people of all abilities are equally valued and safe friendships are made, and where everyone has a chance to explore their talents. From the very beginning we have worked towards live public performances as I felt it was important to give a sense of challenge and reward to people who had not had these experiences before. We soon saw how exciting it was to look forward to our performances and receive applause from the audience, and how quickly everyone began to grow in confidence as performers. Local people came to watch our shows and soon adopted us. They even seem proud of us.

Since then, over the last nearly twenty years, Blue Apple has taken people who happened to have learning disabilities, who had never before performed on public stages, and enabled them to become semi-professional actors and dancers. Along the way we identified and encouraged their skills and talents, building their confidence as independent people who made a contribution to their community. Some of our actors and dancers have toured their performances internationally.

'To be, or not to be' – that is what Blue Apple Theatre and Tommy's whole career have been all about – to enable people TO BE the brilliant, fulfilled and happy beings they are meant to be. That is why our production of *Hamlet*, which we toured in 2012, shines out in my mind. It sums things up for me.

Blue Apple shows just how fantastic performers who happen to have learning disabilities can be when given purposeful activity which stretches them.

I think this is incredibly exciting. We might be helping to improve their physical and mental health long-term, perhaps even delaying the onset of dementia. We see them learning lines and dance routines simultaneously and loving the challenge of performing. People from whom little has been expected are making us think and laugh through powerful performances in ambitious productions. They now have friends and live much more independently in the community.

They have a sense of purpose, are far more alert and interesting to talk to, and most are in good shape physically!

However, I recognise that setting up Blue Apple Theatre and running it might not have made life easy for Tommy. Yes, he benefited because otherwise there would not have been a theatre company and all the wonderful performance opportunities he so enjoyed, but I was incredibly busy and perhaps I was not able to help him develop his independence in other ways. Also when at Blue Apple, despite being with friends and making new ones, he could never get away from me, his mum!

At the same time, without Tommy there would be no Blue Apple.

I later wrote to Bill Nighy, explaining what we were doing and how exciting it was to see the people taking part in Blue Apple discover their confidence and talents and make friends. He wrote back encouraging us, which was brilliant of him.

I remember the very first Blue Apple rehearsal. I enjoyed that. I literally did not want to go off stage, which was not very helpful for the other people waiting to go on. I always used to find it difficult leaving the stage, because being on stage in a theatre at Blue Apple really is like being at home. I have now learned when to leave the stage, even though it still feels like home.

Barbara Garfath, a drama teacher, was leading the rehearsal and in order to get to know everyone she asked each person in turn to simply go up the steps onto the stage and say their name. Some people found that quite difficult, but you and one other person loved being on stage so much you just stayed up there. Barbara really understood you all and where you were, and how to build up everyone's confidence. At the same time, her son, Alex, was generously helping me design our logo and create the first Blue Apple website.

We decided to call our first show *Born to Be Blue*. I suggested that title because we really were born to be blue at that time. We were a mixture of people who had often been feeling sad and lonely, but were starting to be born into the Blue Apple kind of blue, which is a happy place.

I reckon Blue Apple is really important because it gives people the chance to express themselves and to feel the emotions of their character. They should also be able to feel free on a stage. And being in Blue Apple is like being in a family. People make really good friends for life and share their gifts with the world. It is a place where people can act, dance and sing. Before Blue Apple, they could not do all of this. I don't think there are many companies like Blue Apple Theatre.

A few facts – Blue Apple Theatre:

- was founded in 2005.

- won the Peace Child International Rediscover Your Heart Award in 2009.

- won the Queen's Award for Voluntary Service in 2012.

- its first UK tour was the production of *Hamlet* in 2012.

- its first overseas tours were in 2018 and 2022.

I have performed in about thirty-nine productions for Blue Apple in total, including touring plays, dance performances and films. One of the dance pieces was called 'Rediscover your Heart'. It was all about life being meaningless unless you rediscover your heart and reach out to other people. It was choreographed with our dance leader, Jo Tarr, and we were invited to perform it in London. This was Blue Apple's first trip to the city and my friend James went down the wrong escalator, which was quite hilarious. I literally thought to myself, what on earth is he playing at.

This was really early on in the life of Blue Apple. We had won the Peace Child International Rediscover Your Heart Award for changing the way people see and understand learning disability, and been invited to perform a dance at the award ceremony at the King's Fund in London. You and the others were performing to high-profile people like Jane Goodall and other influencers, even, I was told, a princess.

It was still unusual to see any kind of public performance by people with Down syndrome and other learning disabilities so I was keen to gauge the audience reaction.

When it was time for the performance, I moved to the back of the hall to see what happened. Jo and I had choreographed it so that the dancers remained still until touched, and then moved into a beautiful ensemble piece. Jo had chosen perfect music. It was all very moving, and when the audience stayed silent then gradually rose from their

seats to give you a standing ovation, I couldn't keep the
tears back.

I think we all enjoyed performing in London.

You also performed this dance in Winchester Cathedral, at
a national Mencap conference and in the beautiful water
meadows. In every case audiences seemed transfixed
and moved by the dance and by you, the dancers. Jo
choreographed several other dances for Blue Apple, and
we took some of them to the Boomtown Music Festival. It
was a really hot day the first time we went. The grass was
dry so you danced outside the tent. The day was perfect
and people sat on the grass watching. Next time it had been
raining and there was mud everywhere.

I have lots of highlights from my time in Blue Apple.
Hamlet is up there and *The Government Inspector*,
which is a play by Gogol adapted by my brother and
directed by Peter Clerke, Blue Apple's artistic director
at the time.

Pete is an experienced professional director, used to
working with very large casts. Amazingly, he commuted
weekly to us from Scotland for a while. Laid back, with a
strong Scottish accent, he seemed completely unphased by

directing a cast of up to forty people rehearsing together; people with a very wide range of physical and intellectual ability. Some had very few words; some would love playing Shakespeare. Pete knew how to pull together a professional backstage team and get a play ready for the first night. I could rely on him to discover and showcase the talents of each member of the cast.

In *The Government Inspector* I played the Mayor and had to wear a cocked hat with a feather in it. There is something about the hats people have given me for the roles I've played. At least it wasn't donkey ears, like the ones I had to wear as Bottom in *A Midsummer Night's Dream*. I also had a good but battered old bowler hat for playing Vladimir in *Waiting for Godot* and a yellow hard hat for my role in *Casualty*. My favourite was the bowler hat.

Once I nicked Sir Mark Rylance's hat for a few moments when we were performing the Pop-up Shakespeare at the Natural History Museum. He didn't seem to mind. Maybe that was my favourite hat, actually!

Back to *The Government Inspector* at Blue Apple. We invited five different local mayors to watch one of the performances. It must have been quite fun for them to watch, and it was certainly fun for me to play in it. My character was hilarious and I enjoyed it. At the end our own mayor, Cllr Barry Lipscombe, couldn't stop himself coming on stage and giving me a hug. One of the other mayors was in a wheelchair and he got stuck in the lift. That lift was a law unto itself, and it was pretty embarrassing for him and for us. But he did get freed in time to watch our performance.

By this time, Blue Apple was starting to fulfil its mission of giving actors with learning disabilities real opportunities to perform on a public stage. With you as a catalyst, and your confidence and experience enabling others to grow as performers too, we could accept commissions, and push for ever more demanding roles. We produced the play *Freddie's Story* for the NHS in 2008, which was then commissioned as a film, partly funded by Mencap, to use in their Death by Indifference campaign.

Freddie's Story was written and directed by my brother Will and was shown in hospitals throughout England to train medical staff. This was also the beginning of my direct campaigning to improve conditions for people with learning disabilities. It is about diagnostic overshadowing, where a junior doctor ignores Freddie's symptoms and blames everything on him having Down syndrome. It's also about how medical staff sometimes make choices about us instead of listening to us. The nurse asks if it is worth doing Freddie's operation, but the consultant points to all Freddie's cards to show how much people love him. His cards come from his football team, his girlfriend and his theatre company, so he was a bit like me in real life.

Playing Bottom in *A Midsummer Night's Dream* was another highlight. My brother Will, who was our first professional writer, adapted the play for us and Pete directed it. We performed it over five nights in midsummer 2010, when it was very hot and sunny. I quite enjoyed my costume. Bottom is a weaver, but he gets transformed by magic into a donkey. I was not sure about the donkey ears at first, but I did enjoy wearing them in the end. I also wore a road mender's luminous jacket, as Bottom and his friends, who are known in the play as 'the mechanicals', were supposed to be workmen.

We were so lucky with the weather for that run. They were true midsummer sunny evenings. Pete brought in a wonderful designer, Sue Houser, who created beautiful

costumes for Titania, Puck and the other characters. It was
a promenade performance and moved from a grassy slope
into a car park, where we had created Titania's fairy bower
in a dormobile, then into the theatre foyer, the dance studio
and finally onto the stage. It was a truly memorable sell-out
production, too. So many more people wanted to see the
play that they were happy to pay half price for tickets just to
watch the outdoor scenes.

Bottom is a comedy role and I do enjoy making
people laugh. He is quite confident and thinks of
himself as a great actor. When his friends are
planning to put on a play called *Pyramus and Thisbe*,
he offers to take on all of the roles. That is truly
hilarious to play. His friend Peter Quince, who is a
carpenter, gets quite annoyed with him!

Unfortunately Bottom meets Oberon, King of the
Fairies, who decides to play a trick on his wife,
Titania, who is Queen of the Fairies. So he turns
Bottom into a donkey and then gives Titania a magic
potion so that she falls in love with the first thing she
sees when she wakes up, which happens to be the
donkey, Bottom. It is quite a weird and wicked story,
but it was fun to play. Bottom has to cuddle up to

Titania, who was played by Amy, who is beautiful. She also has Down syndrome. I enjoyed those scenes and all the rest of the play.

My favourite speech as Bottom is when he wakes up from being a donkey and tries to explain to his friends what happened to him. I had to stand on a sofa in the dance studio and say:

> The eye of man hath not heard,
> The ear of man hath not seen,
> The hand of man cannot taste
> What a dream I have had.
> It shall be called Bottom's dream
> Because it has no bottom.

Having performed *A Midsummer Night's Dream* we wanted to try another of Shakespeare's plays, and we had an inkling that it might be the most famous play of all: *Hamlet*. That was a big role to think about. Before that, though, I had already started my move from stage to screen.

Chapter 8

Climbing my first mountain

Let's jump back to 2006, while Blue Apple was
starting to get established. I had the chance to
audition for a TV drama. *Coming Down the Mountain*
was my first main audition and I remember it quite
well. I don't think I was scared that day. I think I was
looking forward to it at that point, in fact. There were
so many people there waiting to audition that we had
to sit on the stairs for a long time. I knew a bit about
the story. Jill Trevellick, the casting director, was really
friendly and we did a couple of scenes and talked
about going on holiday, our travels and climbing
mountains. I told her I had been born in the Lake
District.

There were two more rounds of auditions where I read lines and did some improvisation. Once they had a shortlist, they had to find two actors who looked like brothers. In the end they cast Nicholas Hoult and me, but they were worried that he was so tall it would not look right. Then they met my brother, who is also very tall, so they agreed it was reasonable. I didn't know much about Nicholas at the time. He was in *Skins*, which I hadn't watched, but we did watch *About a Boy*, where he was brilliant, playing opposite Hugh Grant. When I actually met Nicholas for the first time he was friendly and kind. He was worried about me being upset about some of the scenes in the film, so we tried out one of the rough scenes and then he gave me a hug. I did feel a bit uncertain at first about that scene, and it was a little difficult to film, but it put me in the right place to react.

I had already learned that acting is not real in my first play, when I played Adam, the character who wanted to be a chef. He had to shout at his mum, and I didn't want to do that. So my mum talked to me about *EastEnders* and the other soaps and the difference between home life and the story on screen.

I remember how I felt when Roanna Benn, the producer of
Coming Down the Mountain, called to say you had the role.
As ever you remained calm and surprisingly matter-of-fact,
but I think you were very happy. I walked into the kitchen
so full of emotion that I could not speak, with tears pricking
my eyes and shivers down my spine. It was your first big
professional role and it was so wonderful that people
believed in you. They had seen your talent and wanted to
give you such an incredible opportunity. You were going to
be the first actor with Down syndrome to play a lead in a
primetime film on television. There had never been anyone
else with Down syndrome in such a role before. In fact I
don't think I had ever seen anyone with Down syndrome on
television at all before.

We filmed *Coming Down the Mountain* in 2007. It
is a story about two brothers getting to know each
other. The brothers are played by me as Ben and by
Nicholas Hoult as David. Neil Dudgeon and Julia
Ford play our parents. I was twenty-one years old
when I filmed this, although my character was meant
to be younger. People have often said I look younger
than my actual age. It was my first professional role in
TV or film, and it was a ninety-minute drama for BBC
One.

In David's eyes I, as Ben, might have been a bit over-protected by our parents. David has to do lots of chores looking after Ben. He gets to feel a bit suicidal and then, when their parents decide to move to Matlock, away from David's school and away from David's girlfriend, for Ben's sake, David starts to plan to get rid of Ben.

He kidnaps him and they hitch a lift to Snowdonia, go camping and climb a mountain. David plans to push Ben off the mountain, but he then starts to realise he cannot go ahead with it. However, in the end he really does push Ben off the mountain and that is the beginning of... but I won't tell you anything more yet. You have to watch the film to find out.

I was looking forward to making a film. When you do end up watching it you might have to make up your own mind about what that was like. I think the story is wicked, and it was fun to be part of something that felt so important. It was important because everyone thought Ben needed protecting, but Ben was quite cool and in fact he had a girlfriend and knew what he wanted out of life and what he wanted to do for a job. He also enjoyed having a laugh, and teasing his brother quite a bit.

I think Ben goes through mixed emotions. Sometimes he is scared and sometimes he is larking about and it was truly wicked and fun playing a character like this. Just a few days ago, as I write, a person came up to me at a service station and mentioned that he saw me in the film, but it is now sixteen years since it was on TV.

Usually during filming they do tend to start at the very end. In *Coming Down the Mountain*, the first scene we shot on the hillside was the last scene in the film.

I remember that first day of filming, walking with you round the corner onto that hillside, and suddenly we saw about a hundred people all dressed in black. There was so much kit: cameras, microphones, huge sheets reflecting light, producers, directors, makeup artists, costume designers, the director of photography and his crew, the sound director and his crew, the lighting crew, and I thought 'Wow, all these people are depending on Tommy to pull this off so that they can make a film.' It was your first film, your first big set, and, as I was later told, no one knew whether you could pull it off. But they gave you this wonderful opportunity and you certainly rose to the challenge. I remember feeling that no one realised what a miracle it all was – you were so professional, working so hard, battling tiredness, building

77

up your filming stamina, being in character, making some of the viewers cry and, best of all, having so much fun telling the story and working as a professional with other professionals.

I actually did feel confident walking onto the set because I do not tend to get nervous that much when I am acting. I really was looking forward to teasing Nicholas Hoult's character in that scene and it was one of my favourite scenes to do. We were sitting on the hillside. Nicholas was drawing cows and I was a bit sheepish, joking with him about his drawing. I had to say 'That cow looks a bit wonky.' I could hardly stop laughing when I said that.

The teasing was fun. I also enjoyed the shouting scenes, especially when I had to shout at Nicholas's character and say 'You tried to kill me, go on... hit me.' That particular line was one of my many favourites, because I was playing someone who was standing up for himself. He was the strongest person in that scene. It made me feel powerful and that felt good. I've done quite a bit of shouting in films since then and also a lot of silence. I like silence in films because it makes people think and feel things for themselves.

 In the first part of the story Nicholas as David had to shout a lot at me as Ben. Nicholas was worried about upsetting me. In the end I had to tell Nicholas not to worry because I didn't mind him shouting at me. I knew it was not real even if he came on quite strong.

There was a lot of teasing in the storyline even though Nicholas's character was trying to kill my character. There was also some romance and a kiss and smoking. I even had to tickle Nicholas in the face with some long grass. So that was all fun, but in real life smoking is one thing I truly hate. The main reason is that it can be really bad for your own health. I don't want people to make themselves ill, because they do have a life to live and they should be able to live it to the full.

We also had fun off set. One day we found some light sabres behind a sofa in the green room so we were having a laugh and larking about with those. Nicholas had been filming *Skins* for TV at the time and he was fun to be around.

Another time, between scenes, I did some arm wrestling with the stunt coordinator. We locked hands. You have to use your wrist and arm muscles, and whoever is stronger wins. On this occasion she was strong, and she won the first round, but I won the second time after pushing hard and getting her hand onto the table. I think have quite strong muscles, actually.

I brought my *QI* fact book along to entertain myself with, and some of the facts were intriguing for people in the cast and crew. I do remember some facts, like Prince Philip was born on a kitchen table in Cyprus, and which is the tallest mountain in the world – answer coming later! Some of the facts might be unexpected and others can be quite surprising. One fact you might like is that the smallest bird in the world is the bee hummingbird, which weighs less than two grams and is just over six centimetres long. That seems quite long for the smallest bird in the world, but that might be the feathers.

One day, when we were filming a close-up, I was sitting round the table with Nicholas Hoult, Neil Dudgeon and Julia Ford and teasing them and the crew with facts from my fact book. Then they started to measure the distance from the camera to my nose so that they could get the focus right. I do have a tendency to make people laugh a bit too much, and this was too hard to resist. I began playing with the tape and wiggling it, making the crew laugh too.

The first week filming *Coming Down the Mountain* had gone pretty well. It had been freezing-cold, boiling-hot and stressful, but other than that it was all good.

One day Mark Haddon came to watch the filming. He wrote *Coming Down the Mountain* and *The Curious Incident of the Dog in the Night-Time*. I really enjoyed working on his film and he truly did understand about living with Down syndrome, and people not believing we can do things when in fact we can. We just need the chance to show off our skills and talents. In the story Nicholas's character sees this, and tries to get their parents to see it too. There is a big shouting scene, and they do finally listen. My character finally tells them he has a girlfriend and he gets to invite her to tea.

Filming *Coming Down the Mountain* took about a month and was quite intense. I think by the third week we were

both very tired. You were still quite young and this was your
first film, plus you were playing one of the lead roles. My
job was to make sure you were on top form. That meant
making sure you had supper as early as possible and
an early night, though that depended, as always, on the
shooting schedule and whether they needed to film a night
scene. I was also the one to wake you up, since you hate
alarms. So my day was even longer than yours, but it was
worth it to show a character with Down syndrome with a
cheeky personality and a sense of fun, his own opinions and
his own dreams. He even had a girlfriend his family knew
nothing about!

Between scenes, or while they were changing the cameras
round for a different shot, we would run lines and talk
about how your character, Ben, was feeling. While you were
filming I usually watched the monitor to make sure you
understood what the director, Julie Anne Robinson, was
asking for in the scene. Do you remember how lovely and
gentle she was? But most of all it was so exciting, sitting
with Roanna Benn, the producer, and seeing you work
like anyone else, getting thoroughly into Ben's lively and
sometimes quite cheeky character. I couldn't take my eyes
off the monitor!

I quite enjoyed learning my lines. We sat in the garden whenever we could so that we were not disturbed, and Mum played the other characters. I liked the story and really enjoyed the message my character was giving. That helped me remember lines, and seeing the lines on the page also helps me learn them.

It was hilarious when I, as Ben, went into the bathroom while Nicholas, as David, was on the toilet to tell him we were going to move house. Not only was he justified in being shocked, I think he might also have been quite jealous of my character. David might have made a good point when he was so angry, because in the story absolutely everything the parents did was all about Ben. It was also not a pleasant thing to hear while you are on the toilet. It might not have been pleasant for Nicholas when I came into the room. He might have felt quite embarrassed when we did that scene, but for me it was kind of fun to play.

There were many highlights during filming *Coming Down the Mountain*, which included shouting at Neil Dudgeon and Nicholas Hoult, something I took much pride in doing apparently. Ben had to yell at David because he had tried to kill my character off by pushing me off Mount Snowdon. And later I had to shout down Neil and tell him to 'Stop shouting, stop shouting', all because my character really was the strong person in that particular scene.

Another one of my personal highlights was talking about sex with Nicholas Hoult. We were sitting in character by our camp fire outside our tent, all wrapped up in our anoraks. It was nice and warm, and a relaxing and funny scene. In fact it was too warm, because afterwards, while we were filming a scene in the tent, I literally fell into a deep sleep.

The clue in the phrase is 'a deep sleep', because none of the cast and crew could wake me up. It was quite a risk filming that scene because there was every chance I would go to sleep within takes, not even between takes. I was in my anorak inside a sleeping bag inside a tent inside a studio, so it really was like living in an Aga on fire.

There were other scenes when it got very warm, like just before I got pushed off the mountain. That morning it had been snowing, but when it came to the throwing-me-off-the-mountain scene it was really hot.

My makeup artist had a large umbrella and tried to give me some shade because I was wearing all my clothes plus the red anorak on top, so I was nearly melting.

Being pushed off the mountain was wicked and also not quite so wicked. It was a wicked storyline because it made Nicholas Hoult's character feel guilty with all the pain he put my character through. There is one particular favourite line of mine, which is basically true: 'I'm the king of the world.' My character felt like that standing on top of a beautiful mountain. I feel like that when I stand on top of a mountain too.

It was quite interesting filming that scene. I was at the top of a cliff with my arms in the air, really happy, shouting, 'I'm the king of the world.' That line was one way of winding up Nicholas's character to really get on his nerves, and it worked. It was the trigger for David to get mad and push Ben over the edge. Hence the title *Coming Down the Mountain*, quite literally.

I had a soft landing, though. It was on to a crash mat.

I remember that very well too. The crash mat was not very big and it was right on the edge of the cliff, which was high and steep. I had visions of you falling straight over the side.

And it wasn't just me who felt like that. When we watched the film with your youth group they screamed in alarm. It all looked so real!

It was reassuring having a stunt double. He had to go over the edge and lie on a small ledge, and then the rescue helicopter that Nicholas's character called for came. Actually I sat in that same helicopter, in front of the controls, when it was on the ground.

I remember most scenes that we filmed on that mountain. One scene truly was like living in a freezer in the North Pole. We had to climb up this rocky path with big boulders, but it was snowing and icy so we had to go carefully. I had hand warmers in my pockets and foot warmers in my shoes and every time we stopped filming you gave me one of the warm coats to wear over my wet anorak!

Do you remember the little train?

How could I not? That was the mode of transport for going up the mountain with all the cameras and other kit and, most importantly, lunch. That was nice as well, having a hot lunch up the mountain.

One day when we were in Snowdonia we had a day off. We went into a little shop to get postcards and a present to take home, but all I could find was a Welsh phrase book. My makeup artist was Welsh and I am a quarter Welsh so she said she would teach me to speak Welsh. So I learned *'iechyd da'* (sounds like yacky da), which means 'cheers', and *'bore da'*, which means 'good morning', and *'diolch'*, which means 'thank you'. I take great pride in being part Welsh. Like I said, I think that is where I get my singing voice from.

We had early starts each morning, so we had several ways of making sure you had enough energy to last the day. You ate as soon as we broke for lunch so that you had time for a sleep. Your trailer was part of what is called a 'threeway'. This is a truck with three compartments for three different actors – and yours had a sofa where you could rest and its own toilet so that there was no need to queue. I think you even had a radio and a small TV in your trailer, not that there was much time for either of those on that film.

I expect you remember the singing?

How could I not remember the loud music. I enjoyed that, and singing with the second artistic director,

Jennie Fava, who also worked on *Dr Who*. When she came over, one particular song might have come up, The Kaiser Chiefs' 'Ruby'. Both me and Jennie sang that song at the top of our voices. That became our special song. I might have dedicated that song to her, but I changed the title of that song to 'Jennie'. That actually still is one of my favourite songs.

Do you remember your driver? He had a black Mercedes or BMW with blacked-out windows. That car had something special in the boot. Can you remember what that was?

Oh yes, of course I can. Mars Bars. It was one way of boosting my energy levels. Those Mars Bars saved the day several times when we had a tough scene, like filming when getting wet and freezing-cold. On those days, between scenes, having a Mars Bar could be quite uplifting, but you have to be careful of the sugar rush, or sugar levels in other words, so now I have grapes instead. Having a Mars Bar is literally having the same number of calories as in a loaf of bread, apparently.

When we were on location that car became your green room. Filming in March in Snowdonia could get quite cold, so we would wrap you up and turn the heating up very hot. I remember doing that when you were at the campsite, just before you had to film the scene where you get into a police car. I think you fell asleep and felt quite refreshed afterwards.

That was the very first time I had been in a police car. It was wicked, although I did not have any handcuffs that time. I will tell you about that later when I talk about being in *Line of Duty*.

So I really did have a good time while I was doing *Coming Down the Mountain*, singing my heart out in my trailer. One day, I had my usual filming breakfast – bacon, sausage, baked beans, hash browns. You never know when you might get lunch so I always have a cooked breakfast when filming. Sometimes you get offered another breakfast when you arrive at the film base. That day I might have had an orange juice when we arrived at my trailer.

BUT in the scenes we filmed that day, I had to eat eight Weetabix in the breakfast scene and then fifteen cookies. After lunch I had to eat eight ice creams in a row too for different takes. Talk about healthy eating!

I could have felt rather green then, but I was surprisingly OK. Doing those scenes might have scarred me for life, but the good news is that I still do like having ice cream today.

You weren't used to filming meal scenes then, and no one had told you just to eat a little. You felt you had to finish your food, but for each new take and each new camera angle your bowl had to look full. So they kept giving you more and more and more. This happened again and again and again. I was watching on a monitor, but couldn't see exactly what was happening. Then someone came out all excited and told me 'Tommy's eaten eight Weetabix!' Was this a world record, eight Weetabix in a row and coming out smiling? I was a bit concerned about you. Fortunately they gave you a break before you filmed the cookie scene.

When we finished filming, the crew signed my script. Julie Anne Robinson, the director, wrote that I had done a really good job doing all the filming, and that gave me a warm feeling inside. I do miss the people I worked with then. It was a truly brilliant experience. Julie Anne wrote: 'Words are not enough. Wonderful, wonderful man, wonderful, wonderful actor.' That made me miss them even more.

Then I went home and back to ordinary life with rehearsals for Blue Apple, college and circuit training, but that was not for long because I was invited to film a role in *Holby City*. But more of that later!

When *Coming Down the Mountain* came out on TV it was up against the first showing of a Working Title film called *The Queen*. So we had a ratings war with *The Queen*! *The Queen* actually won in the end, which is not a good result, but I think we all did a really good job of making *Coming Down the Mountain*.

Do you remember how excited the press got? You did lots of interviews and photoshoots. There were huge spreads about you in all the main newspapers, including *The Times*, the *Daily Telegraph*, the *Daily Mail*, the *Observer*, the *Guardian*, various colour magazines and many regional papers, and afterwards the reviews were amazing. I remember particularly a quote about you from your director, Julie Ann: 'spectacularly charismatic...a very skilful actor...makes a tremendous impact on screen'.

It was very reassuring to read the reviews because it was such an important story to tell. Some of them said:

'Jessop's performance broke your heart', Jaci Stephen, *Mail on Sunday*

'I found Jessop absolutely riveting, utterly charming, a remarkable performance', *Saturday Review*, BBC Radio 4.

'An extraordinary performance…a natural performer', *The Stage*.

'Talented, engaging…on a sharp trajectory to celebrity', Frances Hardy, *Daily Mail Weekend*.

'Jessop delivers a performance of huge credibility', *Mail on Sunday* Live.

'Vibrant, magnetic', *Independent Extras*.

I think the media were interested because I might have been the very first person with Down syndrome to appear in a mainstream TV drama. Everyone was really looking forward to *Coming Down the Mountain* being shown on TV, and afterwards some people said it had helped them understand things better. I feel honoured that they felt like that, and to play a part in their lives. Lots of families got in touch with us and said thank you for telling the story and making them think.

Then *Coming Down the Mountain* was nominated for a BAFTA Award, which was pretty wicked.

I remember taking that call from Roanna, your producer. It was winter, a cold winter's day, and I was in the kitchen. I picked up the phone and walked closer to the cooker. I had been baking, so it was the warmest place. Roanna told me that the film had been nominated for a BAFTA Award and they would like you to go to the ceremony with them. I could hardly speak. I was almost in shock. Prickles ran down my spine. It had been so groundbreaking for anyone like you to have the chance to work on such a brilliant project, and to be recognised in this way was incredibly new and wonderful. I took a moment then ran upstairs to tell you, and you were over the moon. You'd watched the BAFTAs on television and now you were going to be there in person.

I felt really pleased and honoured and proud and excited with it all. It was beyond my wildest dreams.

Chapter 9

Spreading my wings on TV

The next thing I filmed was for *Holby City*. This was in 2007, and although it was filmed after *Coming Down the Mountain* it came out about a month before.

That was my first TV drama series and it was a bit nerve-racking, so they invited me in to see round the studio before we filmed anything. I met some of the actors, but got the giggles because I was so excited that I couldn't really say anything. Everything had suddenly become real.

We walked down a long corridor where there was a photo of the whole Holby cast and of the *EastEnders* set in the olden days. Then I met the writer of our episode, Mark Clompus. We had a talk about the story before visiting the ward where we would film.

My character had to have an operation, so they took me to the room where they have the prosthetic body parts laid out. They are made out of latex, which feels like slippery, rubbery plastic. I quite enjoyed that bit. They made me a latex chest and tummy. They tested out my skin colour to make sure the prosthetic would work, which it did in the end. They also had a fake latex chest with a latex heart. I squeezed something to make the heart look as though it was beating, which was wicked.

They are in the same studios as *EastEnders*, at Elstree. Frankly I am a massive *EastEnders* fan. For the hospital scenes that *EastEnders* do they go into the Holby studios. When I was at Holby I was able to visit the *EastEnders* studio and have a look round.

I remember going into the Queen Vic, which was fun, walking through Albert Square and past the market stalls, into Kathy's café. I think the very first family on *EastEnders* was the Beales, and Kathy Beale is Phil Mitchell's wife. We met Cliff Parisi, who used to play Minty, and later, at the BAFTAs, I met Perry Fenwick. He plays Billy Mitchell, who has a child with Down syndrome.

*   *   *

Back to *Holby City*, because I have not been in *EastEnders* yet (even though it has been going on throughout my entire lifetime).

The episode was called 'Old Wounds'. I think my Holby character drank some bleach when he was younger, and he went into the hospital because he needed an operation. As I mentioned earlier, making your own choice is important. Having that operation had to be his choice only. However, my character's mum, played by Fiona Dolman, was worried about the operation in case it went wrong. The surgeon who would operate mentioned that my character could die, or he might not be able to swallow. My character said he understood the risks, but he wanted to go ahead. One of my favourite lines was 'I want to have the operation. It's not up to you.' Not only was it his choice in the story, but I think that making decisions about our own healthcare like this should also be our choice in real life.

In the story I had to flirt with the nurse, who was played by Phoebe Thomas, which was brilliant, my personal highlight from filming *Holby*. Yet another highlight was seeing Patsy Kensit, who came over specially to say hello.

My *Coming Down the Mountain* father, Neil Dudgeon, is the on-screen husband in *Midsomer Murders* of my *Holby City* mother, Fiona Dolman. That is an intriguing coincidence.

My next TV drama was also medical. I was invited to be a guest lead in two episodes of *Casualty*. Filming *Casualty* was intense and they did some rewriting between scenes, but it is all part and parcel of the industry and it doesn't take long to learn new lines.

Holby City shows more operations and *Casualty* has more stunts, and on *Casualty* they really do not do things by half. One of the stunts in my episodes was when my character, Cliff, wanted to cause a power cut to save his dad from having his legs amputated in an operation. One of his lines was 'You don't have to have the operation, Dad.'

That was the second time I had had a stunt double. While he was trying to create the power cut, Cliff got things wrong. He got blown up in the electricity cupboard, and I, as Cliff, had to fall back out into the corridor. Cliff ended up almost blowing up the hospital and then saving the day, despite one of his arms being severely burned.

I had to go to makeup so that they could give me an injury, and they described what they were going to do. I was still quite young, and I think I was scared it would be real. They seemed to have opened up my skin, and my whole forearm was covered in blood pouring out. It looked really gory, but it literally was not real at all. It made me use my arm carefully, as if it really did hurt, so that helped me to be in the moment and really feel what my character was feeling.

Interesting facts:

Holby City was a hospital drama on BBC television for twenty-four years. The last episode was in 2022.

Casualty is the longest-running primetime medical drama series in the world. The first episode was in 1986.

They were both broadcast on BBC One.

I'm not sure you were too pleased about the makeup at first. It was very dramatic and perhaps a little close to the bone! Seeing you being blown up and then having such horrible burns on your arms was quite traumatic for us too.

I might have felt a bit 'armless about it all, but I know it did literally scar my sister for life.

I remember one day you had a call to film at 11 p.m. at night. We planned our day so that you would be on top form for late at night. We arrived at the base to wait in a green room, and fortunately you fell asleep in one of the armchairs. I woke you up in time to have a drink, get changed and be alert for 11 p.m., but then we found out they were still not ready and we had to wait another two hours. In the end you went on set at about 1 a.m. It was a good thing we had your fact book with us. It is amazing how you can pass the time with a fact book.

Oh yes, I remember that. I think that was my very first night shoot except for the camping scene in *Coming Down the Mountain*, when I teased Nicholas's character about sex and girlfriends. Well, yet another part and parcel of the film and TV industry is often having to wait for a long while to go on set. You just have to have something to keep you busy like a wordsearch puzzle, or researching on your phone, or playing a game or reading.

While all this TV work was going on in 2007, my brother Will was filming behind the scenes for our first documentary together. It is called *Tommy's Story*. He followed me onto the sets of *Coming Down the Mountain* and *Holby City*. He filmed outside and inside: in my old room when it was decorated as a castle, which brings back fun memories, on the train when I was carrying a giant fluffy tiger for some reason, into the prosthetics department of *Holby City*, and in my trailer *on Coming Down the Mountain*, where I showed him my six-shooter Western gunfight impression. He and his camera were everywhere! He even came to the press launch of *Coming Down the Mountain*, and he captured the bit when someone asked me how I felt about seeing myself in the film and I said 'I have arrived', which made everyone laugh. I really cannot take Will anywhere without him filming it. He is glued to his camera!

There are a few people I can quite easily unload my feelings onto, who include my brother Will, my mum and dad and my sister. *Tommy's Story* was the first documentary where I could share my feelings on life, what I was thinking about, and my hopes and dreams. I enjoyed making it. There is a killer line in the documentary where I say 'I am proving that people with Down syndrome *can* act, right here, right now.' I really meant it then, and I really mean it now.

I also enjoyed filming with my brother. We really did have a wicked time working on it, and we had a few laughs on the way. It is nice looking back at it now as it brings back good memories. *Tommy's Story* was shown on television on the Community Channel, which is now called Together TV, and it ended up being nominated for a Grierson Award. You can watch it on YouTube!

I've also filmed an episode of *Monroe* with James Nesbitt and Sarah Parish, and an episode of *Doctors*. I do seem to have filmed a lot of hospital dramas, come to think of it.

Talking about television, recently I was invited to be in *Masters of the Air*, which is a television series for Apple TV+ made by Steven Spielberg and Tom Hanks. That was truly wicked.

I have now done quite a bit of television and many short films (which are fun, though not many people see them), but I would like to be in a feature film – maybe a romcom, an adventure or sci-fi movie, because I like to make people laugh, cry, shout and even swear at the screen. I could play any kind of role that people might like to throw my way. I think it is now time for feature films, TV dramas and period TV dramas.

In one of my short films, *Innocence*, my character did something very dramatic. That particular scene was the highlight of filming the storyline, although I did also have to shout at the bad characters several times. I enjoyed doing that.

My *Line of Duty* character was a brilliant role to play too, because he had such strong emotions, but I am still waiting for a meaty TV role where my character saves the day and really makes his presence felt. I am thinking that I will have to write this role myself.

Chapter 10

The play's the thing

I had seen several of Shakespeare's plays at the
Globe Theatre in London, and both David Tennant
and Rory Kinnear as Hamlet. When people suggested
Blue Apple might take on this famous play I was
excited, but I'm not sure I knew exactly what I was
in for. In the end it took five months to put together,
we toured across the south of England in all sorts of
venues, indoors and outdoors, over two months and
performed to over 2,000 people.

One of my reasons for campaigning, and for writing
this book, is exactly what Hamlet talks about in his
infamous speech 'To be, or not to be'.

This has been a metaphor for my campaigning to help people with Down syndrome to live their lives to the full. Here are a few more lines:

To be, or not to be
Well, that is the question
Whether 'tis nobler in the mind to suffer
The slings and arrows of outrageous fortune
Or to take arms against the sea of troubles
And by opposing, end them.

I think this is about a choice to make in life. Whether to live on the good side or just put up with the bad side of life. He is also asking if it might be nobler to suffer in your mind, that means in silence, or better to try to change things and make a difference – to make things better. If there is anything troubling you, don't just worry about it while doing nothing. Do something about it. I also think that if there is anyone on your mind or on your nerves, talk to them or get some help. I'm not only a man on a mission, but a man of action. The clue is in the word 'mission'. I like to talk about things first, and then do something about it afterwards. Hamlet is a bit like me, except I don't kill people.

When I played Hamlet, we were using an adaptation of Shakespeare's text that Will had written specially for us. We spent a long time working together to find the right lines. One of my favourites was 'Whatever else may hap tonight, look through our sad performance and see that we, fools of nature, are wondrous too.' To me this means that everyone has a gift inside them and we should encourage people in what they can do. I want people to stop saying 'You can't'. Say 'You can, and we will help you.'

Thinking about playing Hamlet brings happy thoughts and happy memories, even though Hamlet was insanely, madly worried. He was tormented by trying to work out what he should do.

One way of getting inside a character's mind is to go deep inside your own mind to feel his angst. I had to go deep inside my mind to play Hamlet and feel his powerful emotions. This speech sums it up, really:

Now might I do it pat,
now he is praying
And now I'll do it and so he goes to heaven.
And so I am revenged.

A villain kills my father and for that
I do this same villain send to heaven.
Am I then revenged? No.

How stand I then, that have a father killed,
*   a mother stained, and let all sleep?*
Why to my shame!
Aaah! I do not know. I cannot reason!
Fie upon't; foh! Heaven will direct it.

I enjoyed digging deep for this speech, showing Hamlet's agony and making the audience feel emotional. I think they really did know how Hamlet was feeling.

Hamlet was our most ambitious production so far at Blue Apple. Adapted by William, but still in the original language, it was performed first on tour by six amazing actors, all of whom have learning disabilities. Their journey to this production was a long exploration of text, character, period, history and personal discovery. This was Shakespeare's play speaking for us all in new ways. His words, spoken from the mouths of these actors, brought new and even richer meanings that would make many people cry and cause some to think again about ability, humanity and potential. Some would even come to say 'this was the first time I have ever really understood *Hamlet*'.

We'd been careful, developing things gently. I had not wanted to overreach any of you. We hadn't. We opened a door to something that would be tremendous and you marched through, full of enthusiasm. Working with William and Pete, our artistic director, we had a really impressive team. I knew they could help our actors rise to the challenge of a really ambitious production, starting with writers' workshops with our core cast looking at text, context, historical setting and Elizabethan language.

I remember I really did enjoy learning how to read Shakespeare. It is not really an easy language to learn, so it does take time. Practice makes perfect! He does enjoy playing with words quite a bit. I reckon that's something that I have in common with Shakespeare.

It was our first Arts Council-funded production, and I think one of the first Arts Council-funded projects which starred performers with learning disabilities. The Arts Council officers were excited about the project too and had been helpful with advice about planning our first tour, but the funding application was complicated. We were asking for real money, and we had to approach public theatres with a brand-new idea. They had to trust us, a company they had never met before, trust our idea and trust performers who were new to professional theatre. The actors were new to touring, new to such intense use of Shakespeare's language and new to holding a whole play with such a small cast. They had taken major roles in *A Midsummer Night's Dream*, but that was more of an ensemble production.

We went through several drafts of our funding application, polishing and polishing our ideas and finally, just before Christmas, we had the phone call. The funding was approved!

I had had to find theatres which would book us into their programmes. It was not easy to start with, but our breakthrough came when I had a brilliantly encouraging phone call with the Minack Theatre in Cornwall, who immediately gave us a slot in their spring programme. Having this slot, proving that the Minack trusted our production, helped me enormously with selling in to other theatres. We wanted to perform to the widest possible audiences so our schedule included indoor and outdoor spaces and theatres across the south of England, from the Rose Theatre in Kingston to the Minack. Eventually we even took extracts to a special event at the Globe Theatre in London.

Rehearsals were fun. There were six of us in the touring cast: Lawrie Morris who played Claudius, Katy Francis who played Ophelia, Anna Brisbane as Gertrude, Ros Davies as the ghost and gravedigger, James Elsworthy as Polonius and Laertes, and me as Hamlet. We were already good friends because we had been in lots of Blue Apple plays together. We had some disagreements from time to time, but we worked it all out and in the end it really has to be my personal highlight on stage. We still are very good friends and keep in touch. I don't see them so often now, but one of my friends does keep me updated, especially about how their rehearsals are going. I would like to go back at some point, when there isn't so much filming to be done.

We started by looking at Shakespeare's original script with Will, who was adapting it for us. Some people didn't want anyone to die in the play. They wanted a happy ending. One person, my good friend Lawrie, said you cannot change what Shakespeare wrote. I think Lawrie did make a good point, and it's possibly wise not to be morbid about it all. I can see both sides of the question. The play is about choices in life anyway.

Another member of Blue Apple said she had nightmares and she really did not want to think about people dying. One way of making her happy was to involve singing and dancing, so I decided to take it upon myself to include both of these. She was really excited about the play after that.

This may be where I should touch on my very own love life, which is mostly private. All I will say is that Katy, who played Ophelia, and I were going out. Katy found it very difficult when I, as Hamlet, had to push Ophelia away to protect her. I had to say 'Get thee to a nunnery, we'll have no more marriages, get thee to a nunnery, go, farewell.' I had to be quite fierce as Hamlet was feeling emotional then. I did keep on telling her 'it is not real' to reassure her, but

I can see why she found it so hard. In the end we broke up, but we are still good friends.

Doing Shakespeare is not at all easy for some people, though maybe it was just the characters we were playing. I have to admit it was not too easy a language to learn, and it took longer for some people than others. We also needed time to really understand Shakespeare's language. I certainly enjoyed his stories.

The writing workshops took about six weeks, then Will went off to adapt the script. Eventually we moved into rehearsals. We rehearsed for about six weeks before starting our tour. Mum and Pete Clerke, our director, had found a designer who made the set and our costumes and a lighting designer who were all professional.

I had expected this tour to be special, and we were all excited about visiting Cornwall, the first time our troupe had been away together overnight. But I had never expected that moment at the Minack Theatre to imprint itself so vividly on my mind so powerfully for so long.

With flyers, radio interviews, direct mailing and posters we had built an audience in a place where no one had ever before heard of us, a small company of amazing and wonderful actors who happen to have learning disabilities, performing *Hamlet* in Shakespeare's language. I had given an interview over the phone with a local radio station and those sympathetic broadcasters had opened another door. They thought our story worth broadcasting. The interview had been on air on Radio Cornwall every hour. They helped us build our audience.

When we took *Hamlet* on tour, the highlight was performing at the Minack Theatre. Every single bit of it was a highlight. The Minack is an open-air theatre with the sea behind the stage. It has fixed stone arches and other entrances which were not the same as for our set. So we could not use our whole set, and we had just half a day to relearn our exits and entrances.

When I first saw the Minack I thought to myself, why are there so many stairs? Another thought was whether my legs would hold up and how well Katy would cope. The steps were very steep so I held her hand and we went slowly down.

Talking about playing Hamlet, my costume was wicked. It was designed by Kevin Jenkins. I liked my sword, and the boots too, especially as I had to hide my dagger in one of them.

That Hamlet jacket is really dashing. It looks like leather with chainmail sleeves and has those silver clasps.

The sword fighting was yet another highlight of mine. We had had a session with a real fight director, Paul Benzing, who directed fights for *War Horse*. He taught us different techniques for stage fighting. I also enjoyed the Hamlet and Ophelia dance, which was probably romantic, but Hamlet was feeling mixed emotions: one was passionate love, the other was anger.

The weather was incredibly hot while we were rehearsing and incredibly cold while we were performing. It was so freezing-cold that Katy's skin began turning blue, so we had to throw coats on her between her scenes. The day was like summer and springtime rolled into one.

I will never forget that performance at the Minack Theatre. Tommy opened the play with a huge, melodic and powerful sung 'To be' speech, which certainly woke the audience up. It was one of the most wonderful evenings of my life seeing you, Tommy, centre-stage, a fabulously powerful, tender,

romantic, sad, heart-gripping Hamlet at the Minack. A
miracle. Each person on that stage had come so far, and
you were all spellbinding. You tugged at all our hearts,
and you could have heard a pin drop even there, outside at
the Minack, where people were huddled in duvets to keep
warm.

Katy performed one of most moving dance pieces I have
ever seen. Jo, our choreographer, had developed a truly
beautiful dance with softly subtle music for when Ophelia
dies. Lawrie's performance as Claudius was full of passion
as he knelt and berated himself, for 'my thoughts go up to
heaven'. For a fleeting moment I wondered, when they had
been babies, had anyone expected anything so marvellous
for them? This was a magic moment. I thought back to these
same people years ago when I first met them; when Blue
Apple Theatre first started. They had told me they were
isolated and lonely and had very little that was exciting or
challenging in their lives. That had certainly changed!

I thought even further back to the tiny baby who had
been so ill, who had taken a year to start recognising the
simple sound of a bell, the child of whom so little had been
expected. Yet here you were, a young man, playing Hamlet,
owning one of the greatest roles in world theatre.

As the audience cheered at the end, I turned round and the woman behind me looked at me intensely and nodded. One man had driven two hours to get to our performance after hearing about it on the radio. He just looked at me and said 'Wonderful, wonderful, wonderful.' Of course, being you, Tommy, you enjoyed the applause, bowed, picked up your sword and saluted the audience with a huge grin all over your face.

The audience response really was wonderful.

They said:

> 'Tommy Jessop was a better Hamlet than many I have paid a lot more money to see in the past and the 'What a piece of work' speech took on a whole new dimension and moved me to tears.'

> 'Hamlet's long dialogues had the audience spellbound, made us really care about Hamlet as a character in a way I'd almost given up on. When he appealed to the audience, "Am I a coward?" it never felt more like a genuine question.'

> 'I was enraptured from the opening scene.'

> 'Simply sublime.'

In one scene, as Hamlet, you moved some people to tears as you walked forward and sat down, looked the audience in the eye and said those words.

I remember :

> *Whatever else may hap tonight,*
> *look through our sad performance and see*
> *that we fools of nature are wondrous too*

You could have heard a pin drop. Here you were, speaking these lines for all your friends and peers: '[we] are wondrous too'.

That is really what the theatre company is all about, showcasing what wonderful people you all are, and why it is all worthwhile.

After the tour, in 2012 my friend Lawrie and I were invited by Mark Rylance to take part in his Pop-up Shakespeare with the Globe Theatre as part of the Cultural Olympiad. The way this came about was that my brother Will saw Mark Rylance outside a café in New York. Mark was very involved with the Globe Theatre in London at the time. Will told him about Blue

Apple's *Hamlet*. He remembered and invited me and Lawrie to audition for him and asked us to take part.

The idea was that actors would surprise unsuspecting members of the public by approaching them and then suddenly starting to speak Shakespeare's verse for them. That basically means you can literally pop up anywhere, unexpectedly, and quote some speeches from one of Shakespeare's plays. We popped up all over London, in the Olympic Park, in the Natural History Museum, which was where I borrowed Mark Rylance's special hat for a while, and at Borough Market.

We mingled with the crowds, then suddenly popped up in a mini-scene from one of Shakespeare's plays, acting amongst the crowd as if we were just having an argument or a romantic moment. Lawrie and I had some fun teasing each other as Demetrius and Lysander in a scene from *A Midsummer Night's Dream*. We were fighting over a girl called Helena. I played Demetrius. Lysander, played by Lawrie, challenges Demetrius to follow him and find out who Helena loves most. Demetrius agrees and says 'Follow? Nay, I'll go with thee, cheek by jowl.'

One of the ways I approached people was to say 'Excuse me, please can I ask you a question?', and then when they said yes I would say 'To be, or not to be, that is the question...' and then go on into my speech. It really was brilliant fun and that was the most wonderful, wicked company of actors. It made me more confident about talking to people. One of the people I approached was Jimmy Carr, who we saw by chance in the Olympic Park, and another was the actor Eddie Redmayne in Borough Market!

I got a surprise that day as two people came up to me, supposedly worried about their love life. I listened patiently, but then I suddenly realised they were actors like you, acting too. So I was taken in as well. I think you were surprising other people in the same way. Another woman was really confused. She thought you were lost or really upset about something and tried to find me. She could not take on board that you were just acting! Was this just because you had Down syndrome?

The Globe Theatre is where I performed some of my speeches from *Hamlet*. We were in the Sam Wanamaker Playhouse. I'd been to watch quite a few plays at the Globe. I actually sat at the side of the stage while I was watching *The Tempest* and *The Winter's Tale*, which really was wicked.

So I actually felt really proud and honoured to be on that very stage, giving the infamous speech 'To be, or not to be'. I wore my Hamlet black leather trousers, my Hamlet jacket and my Hamlet boots, which was quite comfy and nice to wear, but I didn't have my sword that time.

This was my final event for Blue Apple Theatre, a celebration in 2015 of Blue Apple's first ten years, with showcase performances. The Sam Wanamaker Playhouse is a smaller, indoor stage at the Globe Theatre in London. If you've never seen the playhouse you should go. Lit with candles, it is just like being in a playhouse three hundred years ago.

In 2013 and 2014 we also enjoyed taking part in Mark Rylance's Sonnet Walks in London. One of my sonnets was actually not very flattering to the girl I was supposed to be in love with:

My mistress' eyes are nothing like the sun;
Coral is far more red than her lips' red;

If snow be white, why then her breasts are dun;
If hairs be wires, black wires grow on her head.
I have seen roses damasked, red and white,
But no such roses see I in her cheeks;
And in some perfumes is there more delight
Than in the breath that from my mistress reeks.
I love to hear her speak, yet well I know
That music hath a far more pleasing sound;
I grant I never saw a goddess go;
My mistress when she walks treads on the ground.
And yet, by heaven, I think my love as rare
As any she belied with false compare.

At Blue Apple we were producing and performing at least two plays a year. In 2013 Will adapted Georges Feydeau's comedy *The Hotel* (originally *Hotel Paradiso*), which we nicknamed *The Hotel du Hanky Panky* for fun. I played M. Paillardin and had to speak a little French.

In other productions I played King Shahrayar in *Tales from the Arabian Nights* in 2014. We had very rich Arabian costumes. In 2015 Blue Apple produced *Much Ado About Nothing*, which was another of my personal highlights, and a play I also enjoyed watching at Stratford. I was cast as Don Pedro. Pranks were played on people, which was hilarious. Benedick and Beatrice tease each other by winding each other up and pretending they hate each other, so my character became a bit of a matchmaker, as well as teasing Benedick for being single. In the end Benedick and Beatrice do realise that they love each other, and we have a happy ending.

Outside Blue Apple Theatre, I think my favourite play was produced by Daniel Vais, the artistic director of Culture Device. Most of my work with Daniel has been dance (more about that later), but he also came up with the idea of putting on a performance of *Waiting for Godot* in March 2018. The clue is in the title of the play. Everyone is waiting, but we don't know who Godot is or what we are really waiting for. It could be death, it could be God or someone called Godot, but I reckon it's hope.

Daniel cast me as Vladimir, Otto Baxter as Estragon, Sam Barnard as Pozzo and Rishard Beckett as Lucky.

Rishard was happy he had the same surname as Samuel Beckett, who wrote the play.

Most of the time there are only two people on stage, with a few added characters thrown in. We rehearsed and performed this at the Hackney Showroom, which fortunately had a good coffee shop next door because we had to work quite hard.

When I first read the play, I thought it was interesting and fun. Some bits were hilarious. I've got a few favourite lines that my character had to say: 'Pull up your trousers.' Brilliant! And 'People are bloody ignorant apes.' Because that's actually true. Some people can be quite bloody. And some people are quite ignorant, and they behave like apes. I think I might have met people like that – teasing each other, and winding people up.

I think some people are ignorant about Down syndrome. They're ignorant about how you live your life with it. People are confused about what it means to have Down syndrome. What does it mean? It means you're extra-special at life.

My third-favourite line is 'Your Worship wishes to assert his prerogatives?' because it's quite sarcastic.

And I can also be a bit sarcastic as well, in life. But I do like to play people that I'm not like, to see how it feels. It's fun to let the emotions flow out. It's fun to play a character that's full of powerful emotions and understand how they might feel.

I think my character, Vladimir, is a bit like me. He seems to think things through, and he can also be a bit philosophical, and thoughtful. And he asks questions, and he likes to take charge. And he sticks up for Lucky, who gets bossed around by the other characters.

My best memories are working with our director Sam Curtis Lindsay from the Hackney Showroom, Daniel, our producer, and the other cast members. Rehearsing with Sam, Otto and Rishard was a fun part. They were colourful characters, to say the least. There was a lot of laughing. Lots of work on moving around the stage. And I like having a conversation on stage, a bit like a tennis match. Like the line in the play, 'Come on, Gogo – return the ball.' I love acting and I work hard. And it's all worth it, in the end, watching it play out on the stage.

We were pleased with the final performance. Most people watching it liked it. In fact, we had a standing ovation.

Culture Device's production of *Waiting for Godot* was inspirational. Hannah Simpson from the *Journal of Beckett Studies* reviewed Tommy's work in a way that captures the essence of his performance:

> Tommy Jessop is a professional actor with Down syndrome, who played Vladimir in the Culture Device *Waiting for Godot*. He's a thoughtful presence in the rehearsal room, quick to respond to the directors' questions about his character's motivation or the script's possible subtext. On stage his nonchalant gravitas commands immediate attention. He weighs his words carefully, pensively, precisely, and they reverberate in the space around him.

> Jessop plays a laconic and angrily pensive Vladimir, a character he describes as being 'philosophical' yet 'full of powerful emotions' (interview, 2020). He spits out the final words of his sentences with an unnerving bitterness: 'It must…be…dead'; 'What are you…insinuating?' a performative rendering that asks the audience

to re-engage with the lived experience of waiting itself, and by itself merits the standing ovation that the play receives on its first performance.

Hannah's book, *Samuel Beckett and Disability Performance*, has now been published and features Tommy and Otto on the cover.

More recently, in 2019, I played Prospero in *The Tempest*. Richard Conlon, now the artistic director for Blue Apple Theatre, directed us. I would describe Richard as a joyful and caring character. *The Tempest* might be my second-favourite Shakespeare play. My costume was a cloak designed by Sonia Tuttiett for East London Textile Arts. East Ham Embroiderers, many of whom have learning disabilities, helped to make the cloak. It was covered in eyes, which was a good 'eyedea'! I think the eyes might have been Prospero's eyes and ears. With his magic he could see what was happening everywhere when he sent Ariel to do his handiwork.

Prospero might be Shakespeare writing about himself, and his magic staff might be Shakespeare's pen, which created all the different worlds in his plays. Prospero conjures up his magic and Shakespeare conjures up his plays. Prospero's final speech is all about getting rid of his magic staff and *The Tempest* was the last play Shakespeare wrote on his own. Maybe Shakespeare knew he was putting down his pen.

My favourite line in our production was at the end:

> Now my charms are all o'erthrown,
> And what strength I have's mine own.

Charms can mean magic, and I think Shakespeare is talking about the magic of storytelling. They say 'the pen is mightier than the sword', and Shakespeare with his pen certainly drew some brilliant pictures and told some powerful stories, but he knew this last play would be the end of his magic.

I have been in thirty-nine stage productions overall, if you count the Sonnet Walks, plus fifteen dance productions, but I can't talk about all of them here!

Shakespeare wrote thirty-eight plays, in addition to all his sonnets. That's massive.

Interesting facts about Shakespeare:

- *Hamlet* is Shakespeare's longest play – almost half as long as this book!

- He wrote on average 22,600 words per play, but *Hamlet* has about 30,000 words.

- The infamous 'To be, or not to be' speech is the longest of Shakespeare's monologues and it consists of thirty-three lines and 262 words. It was a good thing Will had shortened the speech for me and I did not have to speak for that long.

- *A Midsummer Night's Dream* is apparently the most liked of Shakespeare's plays and, so they say, the easiest, so it was a good start for us all at Blue Apple.

Chapter 11

Growing Up Down's (and getting the giggles)

Working with my very own brother, Will Jessop, is really important to me. Will is a writer, director and filmmaker, and not forgetting a brilliant brother. I was his best man when he got married in 2019, which I enjoyed doing. Let's just say that I could have been the next James Bond in my black tuxedo, and I might have been a bit shaken and a tiny bit stirred. One of my roles was keeping the rings safe, which I did a really good job with, actually. And my best man's speech, which made my brother cry, and that made me cry as well because I really do look up to him. He truly is my inspiration, and I do tend to follow his steps in life quite a bit.

He is good company, and he also does not do things by half. He can be a bit of a stickler for getting ready on time when we are filming. But while we were working on *Hamlet*, we really did enjoy making *Growing Up Down's* together.

Growing Up Down's is a documentary we made for the BBC in 2012–13, which was broadcast in 2014. It's all about going behind the scenes of our production and tour of *Hamlet*. My brother also adapted the script, and I really am proud of him for doing that, actually. Will's writers' workshops really helped to introduce the idea of the storyline and Shakespeare's language and customs. We all decided that our *Hamlet* should be in Shakespeare's language and our production should be as he wrote it, but that there should be lighter moments in there as well. Our story ended up with all of us being dead, as Shakespeare wrote it, but our production did have dancing, romance and some comedy in places.

My brother also told me about the story in advance and I got the giggles because of the way he said it.

Will has a certain tone in his voice which really does make people laugh out loud and it set me off. He filmed this for *Growing Up Down's* and I think you can find the giggle clip online. What made me laugh was that, on the one hand, I thought playing Claudius might be good because it would mean I got to have a wife, but on the other it wouldn't be that good because I would end up poisoning my wife...then he gradually told me about everyone else dying too. That was even before Will started telling me about Hamlet.

Will filmed the writers' workshops, the rehearsals and our tour. We both enjoyed the filming and I think my friends enjoyed being filmed as well.

Growing Up Down's was shown on BBC Three, and then on BBC One, and seen around the world. The BBC showed it many times. It had lots of great reviews in the press and lots of people seem to have watched it. I think you might still be able to see it on BBC iPlayer.

Then it was nominated for an International Emmy Award, and Will, my mum and I went to New York for the ceremony. An Emmy Award is a big thing so we were all very excited. It meant that filmmakers all over the world had watched *Growing Up Down's* and voted for it to be nominated.

It really was quite wicked on the aeroplane. The pilot said that we could sit at the front of the plane and visit him in the cockpit. I was a bit peckish at that time and I noticed his sandwich lying there. I picked it up for a joke, but he said I could eat it. So I ate the pilot's lunch, which I quite enjoyed, actually.

Once we landed in New York we went to the hotel to get ready. I wore a tuxedo and black tie and my mum wore a very nice slinky black dress. We started with a reception at the Blue Bar at the Algonquin, but there was a red carpet and lots of photographers waiting for us. They shouted out 'Here my friend, Will and Tommy!' to make us look their way, and the cameras flashed and flashed. It was wicked and fun.

At the reception there were some nibbles and champagne and I had a really good chat with George Takei, and Lord Julian Fellowes, Lady Fellowes and Elizabeth McGovern from *Downton Abbey*. There was a photo booth where we took some crazy happy photos for fun. Lots of people took our photos and wanted autographs.

The main meal was next, and I had a fillet steak, and sat next to the BBC producer.

Filmmakers from all over the world had been voting for the films that were nominated, so that was a bit of a nerve-racking wait to see if we had won. We didn't win, but it was brilliant to be nominated.

After the awards ceremony we had another drinks reception, where we met filmmakers from South Africa, China and all over the world. We were even interviewed live on radio for Hawaii, which I enjoyed.

The next day we went to see Charles Dickens's original manuscript for *A Christmas Carol* in the Morgan Library. That was intriguing, especially as I have played Marley's ghost and Scrooge's nephew in productions of that story.

It was November and there were Christmas trees everywhere. We went to Central Park and then to see *Tosca* at the Metropolitan Opera House. On the last day we had a delicious pizza before trying to get a taxi to the airport. There were no taxis, so we were

a bit worried about catching our plane. Suddenly
a large white limo drove up and asked where we
wanted to go. He offered to take us for the price of a
normal taxi fare, which was really kind.

In November 2014 we were invited to London as William's
guests at the TV Creative Diversity Network awards
ceremony. *Growing Up Down's* had been nominated for
two awards: Best Depiction of Disability on TV and the
Groundbreaking Programme Award, which was the top
award voted for by the public.

We dressed up in our glad rags, and Tommy looked great in
his dark suit, white shirt and red tie. I wore a simple long
black linen dress which has an offset neck.

We arrived in London in good time to enjoy the Southbank
scene, dropping into the Festival Hall to see a pop-up
performance in the foyer. At ITV Centre there was a huge
queue, which seemed odd, but they turned out to be an
audience for another show. We were checked in and given
gold wristbands, and headed upstairs to the reception past
photos of 'celebs'.

The reception was held in a large bar area with a terrace on
one side. Tommy and I dropped off our coats and accepted
huge glasses of prosecco. We had time to look around, but

didn't recognise anyone, so said hello to other people who didn't know anyone either! After a while a PR person from *Holby City* recognised Tommy and introduced him to some of the *Holby* cast, which made his day.

I met the ITV head of drama and the executive producer for *Holby City*. They told me that there was still not enough writing for people like Tommy because many people didn't realise that there were actors like him to play the roles. That was actually seven years after *Coming Down the Mountain* had been nominated for a BAFTA Award and after Tommy had appeared in *Holby City* and *Casualty*.

William had been working late editing for a viewing the next day, but once he arrived we gathered together with the executive producers of *Growing Up Down's* and paraded into the studio to watch the ceremony. The atmosphere suddenly changed as the top people in TV walked in. Warwick Davies arrived as the host, and a musician and some comedians entertained us. Then William leaned over to say he had seen the camera cue sheet and we had not won. So we could relax and simply enjoy being there.

When we got to the Groundbreaking Programme Award, Jonathan Ross and Gok Wan appeared on stage to announce the award and the winner. We were sitting only a few rows from the stage, and it was fun seeing them there in person after watching them on TV.

Suddenly, I heard the words 'And the winner is *Growing Up Down's*.' I shrieked. I couldn't help myself. Tommy and Will had worked so hard on the documentary over such a long period of time, it was just incredible that it was recognised. I stood up to let William past so that he could go on stage and he took Tommy with him. He 'received the award on behalf of the actors featured' and thanked the producers, the BBC and...me, and there I was on screen!

Will spoke about the wonderful actors in *Growing Up Down's* and then said 'Actually, there's one here with me now. My brother Tommy. I don't suppose there's anything you want to say, Tommy?' He passed me the mic and I sang my very best operatic Tom Jones-style 'TO BE!!!' into the microphone, which I do think rather brought the house down. We can be a good double act, us brothers!

We had a photo taken with Jonathan Ross and Gok Wan. Backstage we had a nice chat and I also met Alan Carr, which was quite hilarious. I was pretty happy!

The after-party was warm and friendly. The producers could hardly keep their smiling eyes off Tommy as he gravitated towards the music and so many lovely people said hello. By the end of the evening, Tommy had met actors from *Holby City*, *EastEnders*, *Emmerdale* and *Coronation Street*.

I watched *The Jonathan Ross Show* countless times and I still do watch it even now. It was great to meet him when he presented us with the award for *Growing Up Down's*, and then again at the National Television Awards party when we won the award for *Line of Duty*. He's very tall, like my brother. Talking to tall people can be quite tricky though, because I am only five feet five inches. Jonathan Ross also invited me to be in the audience of his very own show, which was wicked and fun.

Filming with my brother is calming and relaxing and quite energising because we understand each other, love each other and laugh together. We are making our third film while I'm writing this book, and I will tell you more about that later. I had been wondering in the past when my brother would do this again.

139

The downside of filming a documentary is that it can be quite full-on being in front of the camera, and a bit tiring as well. But the upside is that it is enjoyable and intriguing and you get to experience things you never would otherwise.

Chapter 12

Behind the scenes

One intriguing thing about being an actor is learning new skills for the different roles. When I played Hamlet I must say I enjoyed learning about stage fighting. As I mentioned, we had a fight instructor with us, and learned how to slap or hit someone without making contact. He taught us how to pretend you had hit them, and they had to move quickly as if they had been struck. The most important thing is to make eye contact with your fellow actor before you start fighting so you know you are both ready.

We used real swords too. Hamlet has a duel with Laertes. It is all down to how Hamlet treats Ophelia, Laertes' sister, which is quite badly, and leads to her death. Hamlet is so distraught about his uncle Claudius murdering his father and marrying his mother that he pretends to be mad. He says he is going to put on an 'antic disposition', so that Claudius thinks he is harmless and unable to take revenge for his father's death. But it also means he is cruel to Ophelia and sends her away to a nunnery. Perhaps he is trying to protect her. But I think that Ophelia does not see it that way because she really does love Hamlet. She feels Hamlet has betrayed her, so she drowns herself in a river.

Then Laertes, her brother, is so angry and upset that he blames Hamlet for Ophelia's death. He comes after him to get revenge, and we have a sword fight.

For this duel our instructor taught me and James, the actor playing Laertes, about sword fighting, and choreographed a fight for us. We had three rounds of sword fighting, and in the last one Hamlet is winning, so Laertes stabs him in the back with his poisoned sword. That didn't seem fair, really.

That leads me into talking about *Fighter*, a short film in which I played a boxer. After that I followed many boxers on Twitter, like Deontay Wilder and Anthony Joshua. For *Fighter* I trained with British Boxer Ryan Pickard (Junior World silver medal, Youth Commonwealth gold medallist) in a boxing ring at Repton Boys' Club. I learned how you have to be in the shape of a banana so that you do not get hit so much, and how to keep your gloves up high to protect your face. You learn boxing as a dance.

Another one of my personal highlights whilst training for *Fighter* was when I literally got past his gloves and punched Ryan Pickard on the nose. One of my mottos in life is 'expect the unexpected'!

Fighter was written by Guy Bolton and directed by Bugsy Riverbank Steel, who usually directs commercials, so this film is quite stylised and intense to watch, with a very good story.

That is true. I played Fighter, who doesn't have another name, and the story is all about making choices in life and who gets to choose. Fighter is getting ready to go into the ring for a big fight, but his family are divided over whether it is right for him to do it. Only one person stops arguing to ask Fighter himself what he wants to do.

This is a similar story to my episode of *Holby City*, which I have already written about, and where my character wants to decide about his operation himself. I think it is really important to let people with Down syndrome make their own decisions in life.

In the end we don't know what Fighter chooses. Perhaps he fights, perhaps he doesn't. You should watch it on Vimeo and make up your own mind. Its only eight minutes long, but it's a big story. It went on to win Short of the Week at the BFI London Film Festival 2017, which made me feel very proud.

Fighter had some terrific reviews as well, including this one from *UK Film Review*: 'Jessop handles the intense close-ups and close-quarter sequences with ease whilst mounting an increasing intensity to his physical performance which works wonderfully with the building tension.'

Another new skill was learning to fish for a short film with a delightful title, *Little Sh*t*. This is a gentle film about a troubled boy who meets a fisherman who turns his life around. I play the fisherman. This is a short scene in a short film, but it is heart-warming. We filmed it on a river near London on a very hot day. It was so hot we all felt we were beginning to melt.

When I was learning to fish we didn't have a fishing rod. I remember Mum had to find a long cane and tie a string on the end. We practised on our lawn, with Mum trying to show me how to cast gently, getting the 'hook' into the water. Casting is a bit like a half cricket throw. You hold the rod at one end and throw the top end and the line forward so that the end of the line with the hook lands softly on the water and is carried downstream, where you hope you will find a fish.

With some films you never know what will come next. For *Down and Out* I had to learn how to shoplift and pretend to have taken drugs.

Sometimes you have to learn a new accent for a role, too. For my role in the film *Day of the Flowers* I went to a voice coach in London to learn a Glaswegian accent. Then, when I played Terry Boyle in *Line of Duty*, I had to learn a Midlands accent, which I really enjoyed doing.

As well as these new skills, it's important to be able to learn lines. I have a photographic memory, which helps. Funnily enough, I have actually found it quite easy to learn lines.

I remember you sitting in the garden with the script for *Coming Down the Mountain*. You worked so hard and were brilliant at learning the lines. There were a lot, but I think by the end you knew all your lines, your cues and almost the whole script off by heart. We didn't know then that that was not necessary!

I think my very own brain is the script when I am learning lines. It is already thinking about what my next line might be because I am in the character, in their moment, feeling what they are feeling. When I read a new script I try to see how the character is feeling, their emotions and what happens to them, and that feels really exciting and I really look forward to playing them.

Sometimes lines change at the last minute, so I think you've found out it can be worth waiting until a day or two before you film before you fully memorise your lines.

On *Casualty* they were rewriting the lines as you were all filming the scenes because they wanted to tell the story differently. We found a quiet space and relearned everything inside five minutes. I think they were quite impressed. They had said 'Do you think it's fair to ask him? Can he do this?' Well, you did. You showed them and solved their problem for them.

My photographic memory means I do tend to memorise other people's lines, and one of my personal highlights was when I was on *Casualty* and I learned the other actors' lines as well as mine. One really was shocked by how well I knew her lines. Usually we have to wait for the person to say their lines because it might be a dramatic pause. This actor took quite a long while to say her lines, and I was just starting out, so I took it upon myself to prompt her. Even the cameraman didn't expect that to happen. You need patience while waiting. I did wait, but I think I felt sorry for her. I reckon that is why I did it.

I remember that. Everyone gasped and it was as if time stood still. I looked around, people were holding their breath. Could Tommy get away with prompting such an experienced actor?

I think she phased out when she didn't remember her lines. She laughed when I prompted her. Most people laughed with her then and we finished the scene.

Another time, and this was on my first film, I prompted Neil Dudgeon. I think it was during the shouting scene, the one that I really enjoyed. I had to shout at Neil, who was playing my father. He had to shout and I had to stop him shouting. When you shout you can forget your lines. Anyway, it was a wicked scene to play.

When you get a new script you find out about the character's feelings and emotions by looking at their back story and what is coming next. Then you have to put yourself in the character's shoes. It is quite enjoyable finding out what is coming up for the character and getting into their emotions. That is one of the things I love about acting. The other is making the audience feel their emotions. Acting is my greatest passion in life. I do really love making the audience laugh, cry, shout or even start to swear at what is going on. That is a big part of what I love in being an actor.

Sometimes you can show emotion or even humour through just being still, feeling things behind your eyes and seeing how deep you can get. This can show how serious your character's feelings are as well.

Stillness can be really powerful.

I really admire Mark Rylance in his films, and Takehiro Hira in *Giri/Haji* and Robert Pattinson in *The Batman* for the way they use stillness.

Sometimes there might be something physical you can do to show how your character is feeling, like when I was playing Terry in *Line of Duty* and I started shaking my whole body in the interview scene. Being in *Line of Duty* and portraying those deep emotions was a brilliant experience. I'm so glad people enjoyed it – everyone was hooked! It was great to get my teeth around such an important character.

A typical filming day starts with getting up quite early, maybe at 5 a.m., having a really nice shower and going off to have a full English breakfast. For me this might include sausages, bacon, tomatoes, hash browns and baked beans, a refreshing yoghurt and some pineapple and a coffee as well. Then I go through my lines and get ready for the car to pick me up and take me to the filming location. I always enjoy this because I can talk about football with the drivers. Often the car is a black Mercedes with blackout windows. Once it had white leather seats inside.

After a short drive we arrive at the film base. Here there are trailers for the actors and a costume trailer, a makeup trailer and another one for the production office.

A trailer is where you rest between scenes and before filming. It is also where you have your breakfast and lunch and get changed into costume. You have your own toilet and, sometimes, a shower as well. You have to go up steps to go inside, but they are easy to get into.

The cabin might have a fridge and a sink, and once I was lucky and had a TV but it didn't work. There is usually a mirror and a small sofa where you can have a sleep. This can be useful when you need to be more energised, but it would not really be long enough if you are a tall person.

When I arrive on location I go to my trailer and settle in. Someone usually offers me more breakfast. To get through to lunchtime I might have another coffee and a bacon buttie. This is reassuring because you never know when you will have lunch on set. You might have to have lunch at 2 p.m. or 3 p.m. or 4 p.m., which is really quite late, which means you feel quite starving but it really is worth waiting for. I do enjoy the food I'm given while filming. One day it might be fish and chips, another day chicken and then apple crumble, a full English at breakfast time, a banana and a really nice coffee as well. Lunch is your last main meal of the filming day, so it's worth eating up. You never know when you might get your evening meal, because you might film into the night.

They give me time to eat my buttie, then someone will come along to let me know I need to get my costume on. About ten minutes later they will fetch me for hair and makeup. I quite enjoy this, although I do not usually have much makeup to put on except where there is a stunt scene and my character gets injured, like when I played Cliff in *Casualty* or Ben in *Coming Down the Mountain*. The makeup people are usually really friendly so you can sit and chat with them and the other actors, and I enjoy having a laugh with them. This really makes me feel good about myself and ready for the filming day. You have to go to a special trailer which is warm and cosy and has lots of mirrors. Sometimes on a cold day it is the warmest place to go to. They also cut or style your hair. One time it was the best haircut I had ever had.

Sometimes I might have to have my second breakfast in my costume, which can be wicked, but I have to keep the costume clean. Then I'll have a quick look at my script to get in my character's head, feelings and emotions and the driver takes me to the location to start work. Sometimes I'm completely ready but have to wait quite a long time in my trailer to be collected.

To fill the time when I am in my trailer between different scenes I often do some research on the people that I am working with and their upcoming projects on IMDb, which I find intriguing. I also research the football transfer news, BBC news and the birthdays of certain people. When I'm on set, I like finding out more about how the camera works. I do tend to have a laugh with the cast and crew.

It helps to have early nights when you are preparing for a role so that you are fully energised. It is worth the sacrifice! Then you have to eat healthy food like fruit. Strawberries and grapes are not a sacrifice!

As an actor it is important to keep fit and healthy because you have to work long days and sometimes you have to be quite physical too, like when I had to throw a rapist out of the window in the short film *Innocence*. He was heavy.

It is not just actors, though. All people need to be fit and eat a healthy diet. Some treats are good occasionally, especially chocolate brownies or ice cream, but it is not kind just to offer lots of cake. Strawberries make a good treat too and grapes can be energising and tasty to eat. I often take some red grapes with me when I am working.

I exercise twice a week with my dad. Our fitness programme includes weights, cardio, floor exercises, working on my core strength, legs and upper body. This means that I've been able to do the stunts that have sometimes been part of my roles.

Talking about stunt work in my film and TV roles, as well as throwing a rapist out a window I've of course climbed up a mountain and then been thrown off it, been half drowned in a really freezing-cold lake late at night in Northern Ireland in the month of November, and been blown up in a hospital. Some of my stunt work was done by myself and the rest by a stunt double. Recently I've been working with several stuntmen at once, but that is still top-secret!

In one of my radio plays we did some stunts, too. I am well known in my family for climbing up rocks in the Lake District, but I actually did even more climbing for this play.

The radio play is called *The Climb*, and was broadcast on BBC Radio 4 in August 2015. It was written by Andrea Earl. My character, Frankie, is a mad-keen fan of Sherpa Tenzing. He really wants to climb Mount Everest (which is the highest mountain in the world, but not the tallest. Let's find out about that later!), so he decides to climb Blackpool Tower with his friends, Bud, who is three feet six inches and played by Warwick Davis, and John, who is blind and played by Liam O'Carroll. Liam brought his guide dog.

To make things more realistic I had to visit a climbing wall before the recording. I am not very good at looking up, but this is one way of conquering my fears. In the end I enjoyed it.

Pauline Harris, the producer, set up a climbing frame in the studio and we had to climb it while speaking our lines. In the play my character leads the way, but then there is a dramatic moment when he falls. I might well be best known for doing dramatic stuff, and here was another bit of drama.

Working with Warwick Davies was fun. It was one of my personal highlights. We three were laughing a lot during the recording, trying not to fall off. Warwick climbed highest up the frame. I was wearing climbing gloves and I quite enjoyed climbing. It must have been interesting for Liam too as he couldn't see. Pauline was walking round making sure no one fell off while directing us.

Quick fact:

Mount Everest is named after Sir George Everest, a surveyor who was born in Wales, but its Tibetan name is Chomolungma, which means 'Mother Goddess of the World'.

Chapter 13

Try, try and try again

Before you get on to a film or TV set you have to get the part, so you have to audition. I have done countless auditions in my life.

Auditions can be quite enjoyable, actually, because you never know what might come up next!

Auditions can be quick, although when you arrive you might have to wait a while before you go in. And then you only have a few minutes in the audition room itself.

Standing in front of the director and casting director can be scary, even though I do not get scared easily. They usually start with a friendly chat when you get into the room, but then you have to get into character. They might ask you to do the scene two different ways and I am usually up for that and up for any challenges they throw at me. You should always try to be up for a challenge when you enter an audition room. That is the message I would give to anyone who is going for an audition.

Being able to speak up about what your feelings truly are is really important, too. You might be a bit too shy to begin with when you start, but then you might need to come out of your shell a bit more. Quite often they film your audition, and one of the people in the room might read the other parts when you say your lines. That can be reassuring.

Since Covid, we have also been self-taping more audition roles, which means that actors don't need to travel so far for a quick audition. I actually prefer this because when you do auditions face to face you can get nervous. It is not really helpful if you get all embarrassed, and you can forget your lines. You can feel quite rushed, and I do tend to get quite annoyed being rushed. It can make it harder to remember your lines, and more difficult to get into your character and to feel their emotions. Instead, your emotions might take over. That is all part and parcel of going to auditions but that is also a problem with them. Self-taping is more like filming on set. You have time to get into character and feel the right emotions.

So doing self-tape auditions can be even more fun than doing it face to face because you have time to think yourself into your character. You can show your usual self and they can see who you truly are. When you do an audition in person, sometimes you might also stay in your shell and not come out of it and you also hide yourself away because things are so quick and nerve-racking and you can be quite stressed.

But the great advantage of doing an audition in person is that you meet the casting director and sometimes the director and producer themselves. You can ask them questions about the story and the character and you can do your scene more than once to show off your skills. If you get the role you will probably have more than one audition. For *Coming Down the Mountain* I had three in-person auditions.

Tommy, sometimes you get the roles and sometimes they tell us they 'have gone another way'.

Once the audition process is over with, it is probably
wise not to get too upset if you do not get the part,
because you never know what might come up next
in your career. Not getting an audition does not
mean you are a bad actor. There might be all sorts
of reasons. In one week I had feedback from two
auditions. One said I was too old for the role, the
other said I was too young for the role! They both
said nice things about my acting, but they didn't cast
me. I would like to know what goes through a casting
director's and a director's mind and possibly see how
they go about choosing the actors and making the
performance.

With two of my recent audition tapes, the same thing
happened. The casting directors were really pleased
with my performances, but then one production said
they were 'going another way' and not casting any
actor with Down syndrome, and the other said the
story was too dark to cast me in it, so they were
rethinking the story and the casting.

Sometimes the casting director likes the way you do
a scene, but then the top producer says no. It truly
is the story of my life them saying no. They really
should take a chance on me more often. I can show

what I am capable of doing and show how I get into character and make people feel their emotions as well, like I did in *Line of Duty*.

I do know they are really good at what they do, but they should look past the label of Down syndrome and see what the actor or actress truly is capable of doing.

Tommy, you spoke to American actor Zack Gottsagen who was in The Peanut Butter Falcon. What did he say about this?

Zack's main message is, whatever happens, whatever people say, just be yourself. I agree with that. People living with Down syndrome really are quite wise people. I reckon other people should start listening to what we have to say as well. Just take note is my message to the world.

Sometimes at an audition, though, you might find you don't want the role after all. When I auditioned for *Extras* it might have been a lucky escape not to be in it because it felt a bit too personal.

Sometimes you get the part, but at the very end your scenes land up on the cutting room floor even if you have done a good job in your role.

That can happen to any actor and it can be quite disappointing. One of my past roles that really did end up on the cutting room floor was in *The Damned United*. They had to change the storyline in one of the scenes, apparently. So it doesn't mean you did a rubbish job acting, just that in this case someone didn't want that scene in the film.

But on the plus side, I did get to meet Timothy Spall and Michael Sheen in the green room, which was wicked, actually. I remember it was a really small room and we were all squashed together on sofas and chairs. Timothy Spall was really friendly and asked about my films and about football.

I do also have general meetings with casting directors, just to get to know each other. We might discuss our favourite films. Sometimes I meet a director to workshop a story too. This is almost an audition, where you try out characters and storylines and see if you have chemistry with other actors. Once I had to fly to Berlin to work with a writer/director on a kind of fairy tale where I had to act out the story with three beautiful young women. It was a dream role,

but he still had to get funding to make the film! I'm
hoping this works out for him. We did get the chance
to explore part of Berlin, though. We saw Checkpoint
Charlie, danced with some outdoor musicians and
had German sausages and some brilliant pizzas.

When I auditioned for series five of *Line of Duty* I was
on holiday in Namibia. The first time they phoned
up I thought I couldn't make the film dates as I was
going to be away, but then the dates changed. By
then everything had become urgent, so I had to do
two self-tapes and get them sent in overnight. We had
been out all day so I learned the lines, had a shower
and then Mum filmed me on her phone. Luckily there
were not many lines, but I had to think how the
character was feeling. He was not in a good place!

In the second tape I just had to talk about myself, so
I enjoyed having fun with that. Another good thing
about self-taping auditions is that when they want
something about you, yourself, you can make it up on
the spot.

It took ages to send the tapes, maybe four hours,
because the broadband was very slow. Afterwards

Mum went for a walk. It was dark and she heard the lions roar. She said it was like the roar filled every space in the whole world.

We had to keep the dates free, but I didn't know for sure I had the role. When I found out, that was one of my personal highlights. I felt like jumping for joy. I knew *Line of Duty* was one of the biggest shows on TV and I was looking forward to it all.

Chapter 14

Line of Duty

Being on *Line of Duty* was like being on the set of
a James Bond film with the amount of stunt work
involved. It was exhilarating. I do like watching a lot
of dramatic action TV, so it was wicked being in the
dramatic *Line of Duty* scenes, including a car chase
and being nearly drowned.

The first thing I remember seeing was all the police
cars, then we had to walk down what felt like a long,
dark tunnel to the green room and I bumped into
Martin Compston in the tunnel and then I met Vicky
McClure, Kelly Macdonald, Gregory Piper and Perry
Fitzpatrick.

The story was all about bent coppers and seeing how corrupt they are. One of them even tried to murder my character. Gregory Piper played Ryan Pilkington, the bent copper who was so worried my character would tell on him that he tried to kill me by getting another officer to drive me into a lake in a locked car. Gregory is actually a great guy. He kept apologising after the bullying scenes. We had a laugh between those scenes and talked music, Formula 1 and films.

Jed Mercurio directed some of my scenes himself, which was wicked. He was very calm on set and kind and supportive, and I think he is brilliant.

One of the things I remember from *Line of Duty* was seeing you walk on to the set in that blue hooded boiler suit with 'PRISONER' written on the back. That gave me a bit of a shock.

That was for the scene where officers raid Terry's flat and arrest him. You were waiting in a doorway surrounded by armed 'officers' in uniform. It was quite scary in a way, even though I knew they were actors. They were standing tall and silent, not talking to you because everyone had a job to do and had to focus on their roles.

I quite enjoyed that. It helped with being in character and I was with Perry Fitzpatrick, who was playing Chris Lomax, the policeman who was supposed to be arresting me as Terry. We had had a good friendly chat about football and films in the hotel one evening so I already knew him.

Jed asked me to explain the scene to you. He wanted you to walk closely behind Perry so that none of the viewers could work out who they had arrested. Then you climbed into the police car and pulled back your hood. We had a quick glimpse of you, just enough to think 'Hey, was that really Terry Boyle? It can't be!'

I think that was the very first scene that was filmed for series six. Jed directed it himself and I enjoyed working with him. I did not enjoy wearing the handcuffs really, though. I did not mind the prisoner's suit, just the handcuffs. They were pretty uncomfortable and you couldn't do anything with them on, like if you did want to defend yourself. That actually helped me understand how Terry might have been feeling as a real prisoner. He would have been feeling pretty helpless and scared.

My character, Terry Boyle, had a truly terrifying life. He had been framed for a murder, so we had several interrogation scenes which were quite heavy and I had to act upset. Terry had been threatened about speaking to the police and was too scared to tell the truth, but at the same time he was very scared of being convicted of murder. He didn't know what to say. So I had to say 'No comment' all the time.

I think *Line of Duty* is infamous for intense interview scenes, and I loved being in character in them. I like the stillness and acting inside my head to make people feel their emotions, making them laugh or cry or shout out!

I remember when you were filming those interrogation scenes. I think they were using three cameras at the time, but I was watching the close-up on you. Suddenly you started shaking your whole body. I just gasped. You were so convincing.

Ken Horn, the lovely, kind producer, was sitting next to me as we watched on a monitor. He took one look at me to see if I was OK, and then stood up and said 'We've got it.'

When I managed to walk round to the door of the studio to give you a thumbs up, the actors with you, Kelly Macdonald and Vicky McClure, looked shocked too! I did actually feel quite shaky after that. It had been so moving seeing you there, I still had tears in my eyes, but we broke the atmosphere with a joke.

To show that Terry was really terrified I managed to start shaking all over, which got Kelly and Vicky all worried and my mum almost in tears. That truly was a one-take scene, which is what I always aim for, being a one-take wonder. But then we started talking football again and they knew I was all right.

I know we had discussed how Terry was feeling completely terrified at that point in the story while we waited for them to set the cameras for the close-up on you, but how did you do it?

I found it was easy to switch from myself into my character and back in those intense interview scenes. I was having a laugh and joking with Vicky, Perry and Kelly between takes actually. I really enjoy having a laugh with other members of the cast.

People thought you yourself were upset by the hard questioning, but I think you were acting. Were you upset?

No, I really was acting. I enjoyed it. I actually felt truly proud of myself doing it. I thought to myself of all the really tense moments that I have witnessed through our theatre group, when people kick off. So far I have witnessed about three world wars amongst my friends in real life. Thinking about those gave me the emotions to play Terry.

There was quite a bit more tension and drama for Terry Boyle in that series of Line of Duty.

After the interrogation, Terry is meant to be taken back into custody. But instead Ryan Pilkington, the bent copper, diverts their car into a lake to try and get rid of him by drowning him. The filming by the lake was actually in two parts, partly by the lake and partly in the *Game of Thrones* and *Titanic* studios, which had a tank of water as big as a swimming pool. Gregory, playing Ryan, had to nearly drown me, though luckily there was a stunt double on standby. He had to go underwater a lot more than I did, and he turned out to be the very same stunt person that I had on *Coming Down the Mountain*. Apparently he had also sat in front of us on the plane to Belfast, which I did not know at the time!

It was freezing cold in the lake. We filmed the
scene at night in November and it was like being in
Antarctica. At least we had foot warmers and hand
warmers. Afterwards I had two or three hot water
bottles to warm up with and later a big mug of hot
chocolate. I highly recommend hot water bottles and
hot chocolate, two of my favourite things after a scene
like that.

We filmed when it was dark, and it was still pretty
cold even when we were in the studio. I quite enjoyed
swimming up and down in my clothes in the huge
tank of water. The only downside was being drowned
in it. We did lots of takes. I really do not do things
by half. But I don't mind these scenes. It is a wicked
experience. They tell the story, and people always
look after you with warm coats between takes. They
had put up a tent inside the studio with a fire so that I
could change and warm up afterwards. It was really
cosy in that tent.

When I wrote about *Coming Down the Mountain*,
I said it was like living in an aga on fire and in
a freezer in the North Pole all on the same day. I
think the lake scene in *Line of Duty* might have been

even more freezing cold than that, even though in Snowdonia it had been snowing.

Do you remember how muddy everything was?

How could I not remember that. Getting down the slope to the edge of the lake was really slippery. At the lake we filmed Vicky McClure's character dragging my character out of the lake, calling for help and trying to warm me up.

Well, that was fun. We did quite a few takes and I got sopping-wet. They kept pouring more and more water on me. That wasn't helpful for keeping warm, but it did help with the scene.

I did have a nice hug from Vicky. She and I used to talk about football and football teams and film appearances between scenes, especially between the interview scenes. She is pretty keen on football.

In order to do stunt work like this you really do need to exercise. While we were quarantining for three days before I started filming, I taught my very own mum the fitness regime I usually do with my dad. This might include some arm movements to loosen our shoulders, weights, press-ups, floor exercises, side press-ups, bicycle kicks, jumping on the spot and balancing on one leg. Then Mum taught me her regime, Pilates, which I quite enjoyed.

The actual filming of *Line of Duty* started just before Covid hit in 2020. We flew to Belfast to film three times and the last time was that freezing November.

The first week of filming was in March 2020. In Belfast we were able to go out for pizzas and spend time with the other actors. That was quite relaxing, and it was intriguing to find out what they had been up to. Our second week was delayed by the shutdown for Covid, but we did go back to Belfast in September. We had to take Covid tests three days before we left home, wear special face masks on the aeroplane and have another Covid test when we arrived. Then we had to quarantine for three days in the hotel and then have another Covid test. It feels like I should have a new World Record in the *Guinness Book of Records* for taking Covid tests before I could get on set!

While quarantining in the hotel, we went for short walks. My New Year's resolution that year had been to do some more walking, which I didn't break, except that I had hurt my knee kicking a football and could not walk very far. I also took part in a Zoom conference with actors, directors and producers from all over the world in an international meeting for the Portland Film Festival in the USA, which was networked by Comcast NBC Universal to, they said, about thirty million subscribers! I'm not sure they all listened to me! I was talking about my career so far, which was fun to do.

The rest of the time I binge-watched *Giri/Haji* and other films. *Giri/Haji* was an intriguing watch. Kelly Macdonald was in it, along with Takehiro Hira, who played Kenzo, and Will Sharpe, who is an exciting actor and a really lovely guy that I met on *Casualty*.

Our hotel was by the sea. I could see the Titanic Museum from my room, but it was on the other side of the docks. It is really high and looks a bit like the sails of a ship. We decided to try to walk there and went across the bridge towards it, but my knee gave way, which was not really at all helpful. I was tempted to go into the museum, but my knee was hurting so we sat outside in the sun to rest and make my knee work again, then we walked slowly back to the hotel. My knee actually is quite better now.

In November, on our last visit to Belfast for filming, we had to do more Covid tests and more quarantining. The place which I stayed in that time was a flat, where I did some dancing for my very own pleasure. I always enjoy dancing in the kitchen with loud music like Queen, the Beatles, Blind Boys of Alabama, the Rolling Stones or Jimi Hendrix. In Belfast, my mum made some space in the flat into a dance studio and put some music on. I found that particular song, 'Nature Boy', quite emotional and it really was a strange and enchanted dance I did to it. The song really makes me feel alive and want to dance. It's about loving and being loved in return.

It was difficult filming a major TV show during Covid because of all the testing and having to keep people apart when not acting together. We couldn't go out for meals with the other actors or have a chat together over coffee. But on the plus side, they did bring some really nice food to my trailer.

And I also had the pleasure being in Adrian Dunbar's trailer, which was wicked actually. It was the last day of filming and Adrian had finished and gone home.

I really hope a seventh season of *Line of Duty* will be made with another story about Terry Boyle. Some people have asked me whether Terry was 'H', the big bad cop. Obviously I can't tell you anything, but if Jed writes another series, who knows!

'No comment!'

Interesting fact:

The first episode of *Line of Duty* series six was broadcast on World Down Syndrome Day – 21 March 2021. (And I was in it!)

Chapter 15

BAFTA Elevate: opening doors

Sometimes when you meet a filmmaker it is not an audition. It is just to get to know each other. I had the chance to do more of this through BAFTA Elevate. This is a scheme to help actors who face barriers like different ethnicity or disabilities get more TV and film work. They might be actors one year and producers or writers another year. I applied for it because I wanted to break down barriers and make myself heard in the industry, and I was lucky enough to be one of twenty-one people chosen in 2020. I'm truly grateful to everyone who supported my application to make this happen.

BAFTA helped us to develop our careers. They arranged for us to meet famous directors and writers at round-table events and to have one-to-one sessions with casting directors.

The first time I walked through BAFTA's door in Piccadilly, London, had been for the launch of my short film *Innocence*. That was pretty exciting. When I went there for Elevate I was really looking forward to it all.

It was an hour's journey up to London. I did more research on my phone on the train and then had a half-hour walk to BAFTA. When we got there I enjoyed talking to other people on the scheme. They were fun as well, and good company. I would like to work with them, and would be up for a BAFTA reunion! There was some pretty good food before the events too, including sausages, big plates of hummus and flatbreads, crisps and amazing brownies.

One of my personal highlights was meeting Cary Fukunaga. He was making *No Time To Die* at the time, the latest James Bond film, and I truly recommend people to watch if they haven't already done so. We met at a round table at BAFTA with the other Elevate actors.

Later, I was given the small role in *Masters of the Air*. I did not mind at all having a small role. It was truly wicked playing the role and seeing how a big Hollywood film set works. The answer is pretty fast-moving, but that was fine!

Meeting David Yates was yet another one of my personal highlights from the BAFTA Elevate scheme, because he directed some of the *Harry Potter* series, something I do tend to watch quite a lot. We met in a London café and had a good chat about films and football. He was just finishing the edit of *Fantastic Beasts: The Secrets of Dumbledore* so he couldn't give me a role in that, but I did enjoy watching it when he invited me to the premiere in London! David was just off to America to film. Maybe we will have the chance to work together in the future. I hope so, because I watch all of his films on loop.

I also met some brilliant casting directors, including the casting director for James Bond. I was quite shaken, but not stirred, by meeting her. That made her laugh. I went to her house and we had a good chat about my work, about casting and about our favourite James Bond films. *No Time to Die* has to be mine, now. I am also intrigued by how a casting director works, and how they choose the right actors for the roles.

Usually we went to the BAFTA headquarters for the events, which was fun. But during Covid lockdowns I had to meet people one to one on Zoom, including David Heyman, who made the brilliant *Paddington* films and Richard Curtis, who made some of my favourite films, *About Time*, *Yesterday* and *The Boat that Rocked*.

One day in autumn 2022, I was filming in London with my brother before we went to a private BAFTA screening of *Elvis*, which has to be a highlight. There were two reasons for this. The first is because it has Austin Butler playing Elvis, and Tom Hanks in it as well. I had been working in the same series as Austin Butler that had been top-secret for nearly two years. I met Austin outside his trailer and in makeup when I was filming, and we had a good talk about what he had been in lately, about football teams that we support and about American football. He is a really nice person and really good fun.

The *Elvis* screening was at the Ham Yard Hotel. As we were getting ready to watch it and making sure our camera was safe in the left luggage, a familiar voice rang out saying 'Tommy Jessop!' This was the second reason it was a highlight. That particular voice, which was a warming voice, was Richard Curtis.

I am hoping there might be two godparents to my film career. My godfather would be Richard Curtis and my godmother has to be Sally Phillips, who I have loved working with in the past.

I would love to work with Richard in the future. I really like his films because he thinks deeply about his characters and makes you care about them. He has a great imagination. My favourite film he has ever done is *About Time*, which is very emotional. I do enjoy watching emotional films because they really make you think about the characters. I reckon that is one thing I have in common with Richard Curtis — we really do like to make people feel characters' emotions, which is a good thing to happen.

The film *Elvis* was quite emotional too. He really had ups and downs in his life and in his career, and he lived a good life to the full. I also liked listening to the music, which made me want to dance.

At the end of the screening Richard Curtis introduced a Q&A with Baz Luhrmann, who directed the film. I really did enjoy listening to that. One of the most intriguing things I found out was that it took ten years to make the film. That is impressive. Baz Luhrmann wanted to be truthful and really show what Elvis's life was like back then. He mentioned Tom Hanks getting Covid, which held up filming because he did not want to infect other people while making it. He was that ill, apparently. He played Colonel Tom Parker and I thought did a really good job showing what life was like when he was working with Elvis. Colonel Tom Parker was a complicated figure in Elvis's life and he was quite emotional after Elvis's passing. I think Tom Hanks did a good job of showing his conflicting emotions.

Every year BAFTA holds the David Lean Lecture, given by one of the world's best filmmakers. In 2022 it

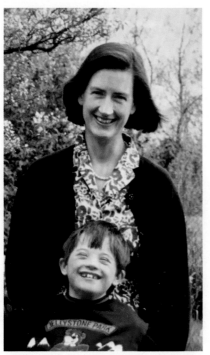

Mum and me having fun in the garden
© Jessop family

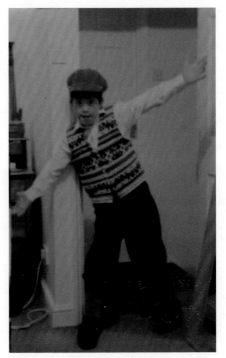

Loving an audience
© Jane Jessop

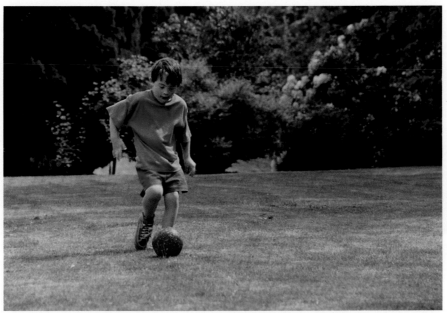

My first dream – to be a professional footballer
© Jessop family

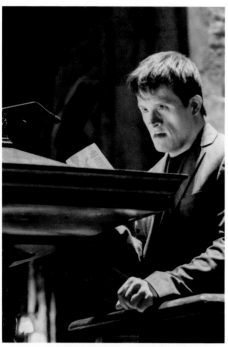

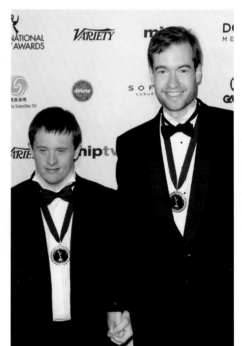

Reading John Betjeman's 'And is it true?' at Mencap's Christmas celebration in the oldest church in London

© Mencap

With my brother, Will, in New York at the International Emmys for our film *Growing Up Downs*

© Everett Collection Inc / Alamy

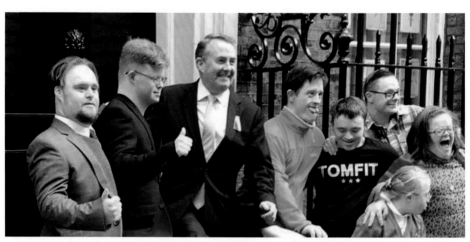

Outside Number 10 with (L to R) Fionn Crombie Angus, Max Ross, Dr Liam Fox MP, Tom Enoch, James Carter, Beth Costerton and Heidi Crowter on World Down Syndrome Day 2022

© Jane Jessop

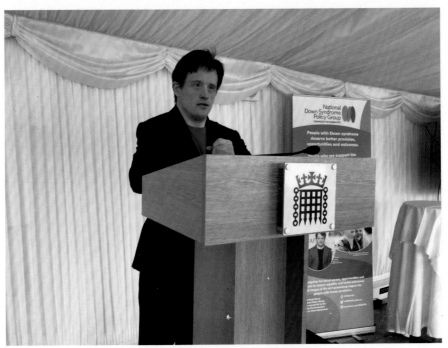

Making our voices heard in Parliament, March 2022
© Jane Jessop

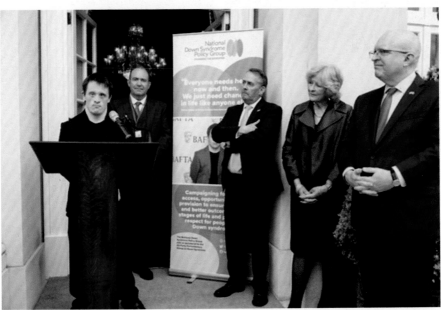

Speaking at the US Embassy, July 2022 (L to R) me, Ken Ross, Dr Liam Fox MP,
Baroness Hollins, US Chargé d'affaires Ambassador Philip Reeker
© National Down Syndrome Policy Group

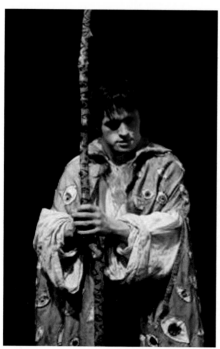

Wearing Prospero's Cloak of Many Eyes
for Blue Apple Theatre's *The Tempest,* 2019
© Mike Hall

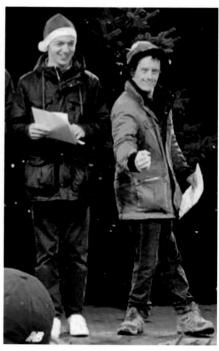

Singing my heart out for Christmas
with the Blue Apple singers
© Jane Jessop

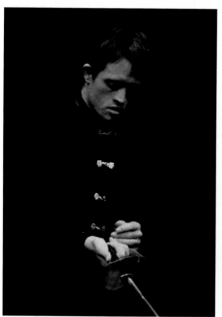

Playing Hamlet: 'To be or not to be?'
That truly is a big question
© Will Jessop

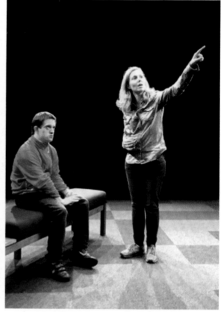

Rehearsing a scratch comedy with
my good friend Sally Phillips at
The Orange Tree Theatre
© Jane Jessop

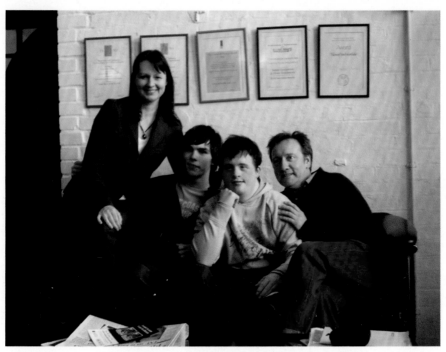

My on-screen family in *Coming Down the Mountain*
(L to R) Julia Ford, Nicholas Hoult, me, Neil Dudgeon
© Jane Jessop

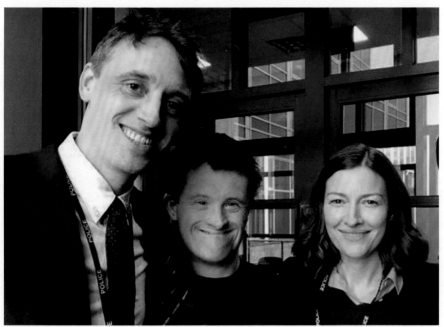

First day at *Line of Duty*: meeting Perry Fitzpatrick and Kelly Macdonald
© Jane Jessop

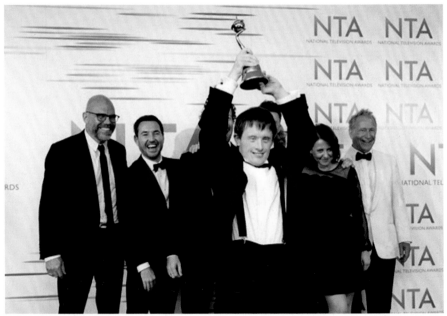

Line of Duty wins again! At the National Television Awards –
I was on cloud 9, on top of the world!

© Ian West/PA Images/Alamy

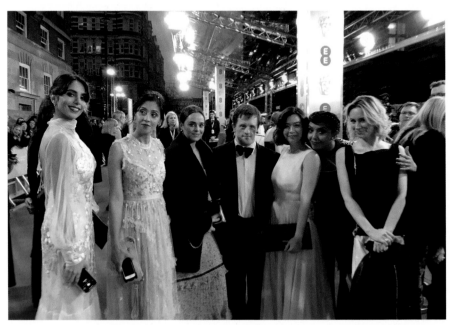

At the BAFTAs with other actors from BAFTA Elevate (L to R) Anjli Mohinder,
Manjinder Virk, Aysha Kala, me, Naomi Yang, Sunetra Sarker and Kellie Shirley

© Jane Jessop

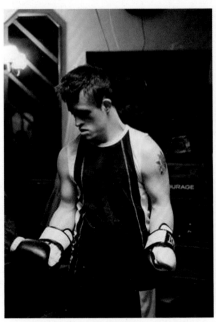

Between scenes filming *Fighter*
© Luke Atkinson

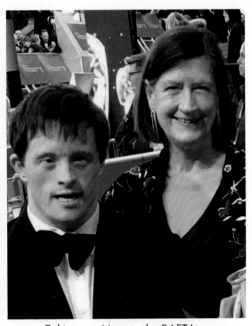

Taking my Mum to the BAFTAs –
who knows what might happen!
© Photo taken on Jane's camera by a passer-by

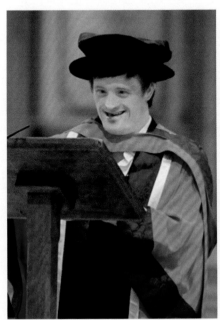

Speaking to students in Winchester
Cathedral after receiving my
Honorary Doctorate of the Arts
© University of Winchester

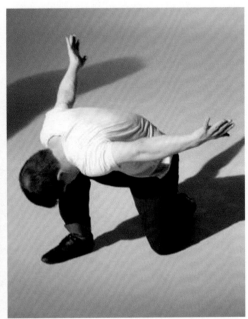

Dancing with Culture Device
© Jane Jessop

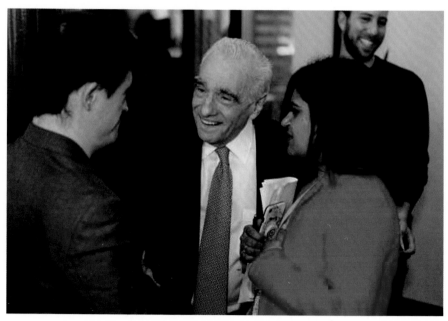

It was absolutely wicked meeting film legend Martin Scorsese
with Mariayah Kaderbhai thanks to BAFTA Elevate

© Jonny Birch/BAFTA via Getty Images

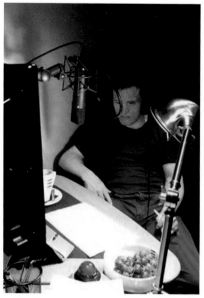

Recording a voiceover for *Panorama*

© Jane Jessop

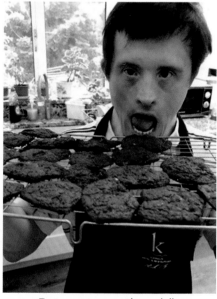

Trying out my cooking skills

© Jane Jessop

was by Ryan Coogler, who is the writer of the *Black Panther* films and *Creed*, which is a spinoff of *Rocky*. This is quite handy because my short film *Fighter* was also set in the world of boxing.

The train journey to London this time was good fun, but it was the month of December, and I wore two coats as it was so cold.

There was champagne and some nibbles when we arrived, and I enjoyed listening to Ryan Coogler's lecture, which was emotional and moving. Ryan described himself as being a black filmmaker, and in the same way I might be a filmmaker with Down syndrome.

It was quite emotional when he talked about Chadwick Boseman's sad passing. To Ryan Coogler himself, Chadwick Boseman really was the Black Panther. Ryan said each film has to be about a question. In *Black Panther: Wakanda Forever*, the question is how do you move on when you lose the hero that defines you? It is all about dealing about grief, and how to move on from it.

Hearing about the *Black Panther* films was particularly intriguing because my dream is to star in my very own superhero film. The main message about making any superhero films really should be getting your story told no matter how emotional you might get telling it, I reckon.

Last but by no means least, meeting Martin Scorsese in October 2019 really was the personal highlight of my time with BAFTA Elevate. I was utterly speechless when I shook his hand after he had given his David Lean Lecture, just before lockdown. We had all gone into the bar to meet people and have a drink. I had to move to the other side of the room as I needed a soft drink, and there he was. I wanted to talk to him about stillness and powerful acting, but, as I said, I was suddenly speechless so we just shook hands and took a long, good, happy look at each other. He was the same height as I am and very smiley and kind.

Now I am a full member of BAFTA, which means I can meet people in the members' bar and go to screenings there. I get to watch a lot of films and television programmes and then vote for them in the BAFTA Awards. That is pretty much my dream job!

Chapter 16

And the winner is...

How about joining me at an award ceremony? Let's start with the RADAR People of the Year Human Rights Media Awards 2008, my very own first award ceremony. I went with Roanna Benn, who produced *Coming Down the Mountain* and who now runs Drama Republic. We dressed up for the awards and had a nice supper at a big round table. *Coming Down the Mountain* won an award so Roanna and I both made speeches, which I really enjoyed.

Since then, I have been to the BAFTA Awards three times, which really is wicked. The very first one that I went to was when *Coming Down the Mountain* was nominated for Best Single Drama in the BAFTA TV Awards.

We had decided to stay at the hotel on the park where the dinner and after-party were held. Dad drove us up to London and Mum and I checked in. I changed into black tie and Mum wore a long floaty dress.

You looked terrific. My hairdresser, the wonderful Guy Kremer, had been so excited for us that he had opened his salon specially that Sunday morning so that he could help us look as glamorous as possible!

The hotel booked us one of those black cars with blacked-out windows, and when we arrived at the London Palladium for the ceremony there was a quite a queue. We waited our turn, and as we pulled up our car was suddenly surrounded by photographers. They were not very interested in me, of course, but cameras flashed continuously at you! We walked slowly down the long red carpet, enjoying the fun and the crowds, mingling with actors, producers, directors and famous faces from the media. Finally, it was your turn to face the tall bank of photographers. You just stood there like a pro as cameras from the world press flashed and flashed and flashed.

I felt I had finally arrived. I think that also might mean I mixed the good emotions of feeling excited to be there with enjoying it all. Every time I mention 'I have arrived', I mean all my dreams have come true.

I rather enjoyed standing there for the photographers. It was a pleasantly warm and exciting feeling to be doing that. Then we went into the London Palladium and found our seats. Heidi Thomas, who created *Call the Midwife*, was sitting just in front of us. That was the first time we met her and it was fun talking to her. We talked about her brother, who had had Down syndrome, but he had died. We also talked about *Coming Down the Mountain*, which she had loved watching. I think she was pleased for me to have that role and to be at the BAFTAs.

When we got to the Best Single Drama category, I felt proud and honoured to be up for that award. Roanna said I should go up on stage if we won, so I had a speech in my head just in case. We didn't win (I reckon we should have), but it was brilliant to be nominated anyway.

Next we went to the dinner and after-party. As we went up the stairs I met Perry Fenwick from

EastEnders, whose character had a baby with Down syndrome. He was really friendly and introduced me to more of the cast. He told me he was named after Perry Como. I also had a chat with Cliff Parisi of *EastEnders*.

Simon Amstell was there – he was the host of *Never Mind the Buzzcocks* then – and the comedian Harry Hill, who is famous for wearing those big collars and who I had a chat with later. I also had a chat with David Mitchell, one half of *Mitchell and Webb*, a show I used to watch.

Piers Morgan was there, and at dinner I sat next to James Nesbitt, which was wicked. I found out which team he supports, which appears to be Manchester United. I think most people up in Northern Ireland do support Man U, apparently. I worked with James Nesbitt later, on *Monroe*, which was an ITV hospital drama. I also enjoyed working with Sarah Parish on that series.

At dinner we sat at round tables with flowers in the middle and all sorts of other decorations. Dame Judi Dench was at the next table. I felt speechless in her presence. Who would not!

At the after-party, I had a chat and a laugh with Harry Hill. I still have his joke book in my room, which I should dig out again. Then I had a good dance with lots of girls while Mum chatted to Nick Hewer from *The Apprentice*. She said they both felt a bit like lemons while all the dancing was going on, but she likes talking business with people anyway, so she was happy.

At midnight I was still dancing. I might be best known as a night owl because I really do come out quite late at night. This is not good news for some people, but for me it is. I do know my limits, and when to turn in for an early night before an audition or any filming that might come my way. But if you are dancing at the BAFTAs you are bound to stay up late at night, especially if my mother is there. If you are around, Mum, you really do make good company for me and for other people, which is reassuring and puts us in a good mood.

The second awards show that I went to was as a BAFTA Elevate member in 2019 at the Royal Albert Hall. This time I sat near the roof, which was brilliant.

And at the third one, in 2020, I presented a TV BAFTA Award for the Best Daytime Show. It was during Covid, so we had to pre-record the videos and then send them in. I didn't know who had won until the night itself, when I watched it on television, so I had to film giving the award to each nominee, one after the other, and they would only use one clip, the one for the winner. It was *The Great House Giveaway*. I really did enjoy it. I thought it was an honour being a part of it all, although I did miss the after-party. However, it was probably wise that I did not go. My very own brother filmed me through the glass doors in my house while I presented the award, which really was wicked. I will let you in on a little secret though, which is that although I was wearing a dinner jacket and bow tie in the video, I was actually wearing green crocs on my feet! They are very comfortable and I felt I was quite a snappy dresser!

It was so exciting when this invitation came through because it was another first. Someone with Down syndrome was on this world stage, and we were all thrilled that it could be you.

*　　*　　*

The Casting Directors' Guild invited me to present an award at their March 2022 annual ceremony. They gave us a hotel and a car to take us to the Ham Yard Hotel for the event. I decided to wear my new green jacket instead of my tuxedo.

We had tried to find out the dress code, and been told no one would wear a tux. Unfortunately it became obvious that one of the casting directors was hoping to have seen you in your tux. As your support and help I felt rather guilty about that.

We walked through the bar area, which was full of tall people and lots of noise of conversation and laughing, and were invited into a room for presenters. There was champagne and lovely food, and we could sit down and talk more easily. It can be quite difficult making yourself heard in a crowded room where people are taller than you are.

I met Jessica Plummer from *EastEnders*, Ncuti Gatwa, who is now playing Dr Who, and James Norton, who is tipped as a possible James Bond if I don't get the role first. They were also presenting awards. I also met casting directors from some very famous films.

This was really affirming, really good fun and pretty exciting, though also nerve-racking. Think how many casting directors would see Tommy in person and, I was hoping, maybe remember him for future roles.

I was presenting with Emily Barber, who was quite nervous, so I reassured her that it's fine if you are a bit nervous, but not too nervous. We swapped stories about our careers, the films and TV we had been in and worked out who would introduce the category and who would announce the winner. Then we went off into the auditorium to rehearse.

We were shown to our seats and watched other people presenting the first awards. At last our moment came. We got up together and moved towards the stage. We had to cross in front of the whole audience in order to reach the steps. Emily waited for me to go up the steps so that we could walk onto the stage together, at least until I couldn't help dancing with excitement, doing my twirling bow. We presented the award for Best Casting in a TV Drama Series, which was won by Cole Edwards, the casting director of *Line of Duty*, who had cast me.

I made a little speech, which I enjoyed delivering.

*   *   *

A few months before this, one day in autumn 2021, we'd had another phone call. It was from the organisers of the National Television Awards. *Line of Duty* had been nominated for the Returning Drama Award and was also going to be honoured with the Special Recognition Award for its ten-year anniversary, and they invited Tommy to attend, with us to support him.

They gave us lovely rooms at the Athenaeum Hotel in Piccadilly, and sent a car to take us to the O2 where the awards were being held. This time I did wear my black-tie tuxedo.

When we arrived I had to walk up the red carpet and talk to the press. I gave a recorded interview for *What's On TV*, which was wicked as I like reading that magazine. Then there were lots of press photographers waiting to photograph everyone as they went in.

Before the ceremony there was a champagne reception where we caught up with the other people from *Line of Duty* and I had another chat with Jonathan Ross. During the evening I met Ant and Dec, Alan Carr again, Michael McIntyre, the producer of the *Great British Bake Off* and Anne Hegerty from *The Chase* (who has two nicknames, The Governess and Frosty Knickers, which is how she introduced herself to us!) and lots of other television stars.

We sat near the front and the ceremony began with a performance from JLS, which was brilliant, especially as we were so close to the stage. We sat in front of the people from *RuPaul's Drag Race*, and I had a really nice chat about Newcastle United football team with Ant and Dec. I had another chat with Olly Alexander, which I really enjoyed.

When they called out *Line of Duty* I jumped up with excitement and full of joy. They had asked me to go on stage with them, so I did. I followed them and that's when I did my big Brucie Pose and everyone laughed and joined in the fun. People stood up and applauded. The other actors were laughing and the pictures were all over the newspapers next day. I just wanted to do something spontaneous and fun to celebrate with everyone and make them laugh.

On 11 June 2022 I presented at the British Soap Awards with Gregory Piper. The award was for Best

Villain, which was quite funny as Gregory had of course played the villain in *Line of Duty*.

We were put up in a hotel in London and they sent a car to take us to Hackney Town Hall for the ceremony. They sent us back at the end of the evening in a lovely new Tesla.

I wore my dark suit and a white shirt with an open collar, no tie for this one as it was a bit less formal. They had put up a tent lined with red curtains for the presenters where there was champagne and small things to eat, although I decided not to have any champagne until after our presentation and then it was all gone! It really was a wicked time there, meeting Barney Walsh from *Breaking Dad* and Connor McIntyre from *Coronation Street* and then having a hug and talking with Janette Manrara and Aljaž Škorjanec from *Strictly Come Dancing* and Esme Young and Patrick Grant, the judges from *The Great British Sewing Bee*. Gregory brought his girlfriend, who was currently in *The Archers* on BBC Radio 4.

We went on stage to rehearse and try out the microphones, and then back to the tent to relax and talk to the others.

Phillip Schofield was the host. When it was our turn, Phillip introduced us by saying 'Here to unmask the wicked winner are two people who have seen their own fair share of foul play and dodgy dealings, just don't tell that to AC-12! From the phenomenal *Line of Duty*, it's Tommy Jessop and Gregory Piper.' We walked on stage and there was a lot of cheering, which I really enjoyed.

There was a pretty glamorous after-party too where I met lots of actors including Danny Dyer, who played Mick Carter in *EastEnders*. They gave each of us presenters a beautiful white orchid. It was quite funny fitting that into the Tesla and taking it home on the train next day.

In 2021 the University of Winchester gave me a different sort of award, one that is a truly great and proud honour in my life. The university made me an Honorary Doctor of Arts, which was wicked.

I am passionate about this because the performing arts really are important for people to learn new skills and discover new ideas through the stories we tell.

I had to wear a long red gown and black floppy hat, and polish up a speech to give in Winchester Cathedral to all the students and their families. I enjoyed processing round the cathedral with Alan Titchmarsh, who was the Chancellor, and Elizabeth Stuart, Vice-Chancellor of the university, and lots of the staff and governors. They were all wearing gowns and floppy hats too, although their gowns had more gold on them than mine.

You had to walk past all the students and their families up the longest cathedral nave in Europe. The cathedral was completely full.

I think I am quite well known for making my presence felt on stage, and that day it was by dancing. The excitement of it all, with everyone clapping, made me dance. I was supposed to bow to Alan Titchmarsh, but I couldn't stop myself dancing, although I did bow in the end. Then someone made a speech about me and that was surprisingly pleasing. Then I made my speech, which was one of the personal highlights in my life. I hope it sent a powerful message to everyone. Hopefully it will inspire those students to follow their dreams, be happy with their lives and be kind people. I told them my dream is to be the next James Bond. Why not?!

I've also received some personal awards for my acting, which is brilliant. The first time I was nominated for a Best Lead Actor Award was at the Southampton Film Festival for my short film *Down and Out*. I won! It was so exciting I could not stop smiling. I had to make a thank you speech, but my smiling kept getting in the way. I was so happy.

Tommy, I'm so proud of you. You have had so many wonderful Best Actor nominations and awards, and your short films have been shown in over fifty festivals around the world. To select just a few: *Down and Out* also won you a Best Actor award at Kinofilm Festival, Manchester, and was officially selected for twenty-two festivals in the UK and US, including the International New York Film Festival.

You won a further Best Actor award at the Oska Bright film Festival for *Fighter*, which also won Best Film at Film London, was selected as Short Of The Week at the BFI London Film Festival and was nominated for Best Film at Chelmsford Film Festival.

You were voted Best Actor at the Suffolk film Festival for *Innocence*, which was also voted Best Short Film at London Lift Off. *Innocence* was shown at thirty film festivals worldwide, winning six prestigious titles, and then longlisted for both a BAFTA and an Oscar!

Of course to be nominated for the International Emmy Award, *Growing Up Down's* must have been shown in even more places around the world.

It is truly exciting every time I am nominated or win an award and I really am grateful for people voting for me.

It's been interesting meeting so many celebrities at these award shows, and also when I'm filming for TV and films. People do recognise me in the street now, and it's made me think about what 'celebrity' means. To me, it does not mean you are any different from before you were a celebrity or from other people, but it does mean fun.

Being a celebrity basically means mingling with all the famous people that you would really want to meet, and drinking champagne. Other really nice people might want you to sign autographs and say thank you for being there and for what you have done in your life and career.

There are some things that are meant to be private, so you have to bear that in mind and keep them secret when you are meeting people or talking to journalists.

A lot of social media comes with celebrity, as well as being interviewed for the papers and being on the radio and TV.

And it might make your journeys easier when you're sent a chauffeur-driven Tesla.

Sometimes, though, the attention can be a bit too much. One day I was on set filming *Masters of the Air*, the Steven Spielberg TV series which at the time was very hush-hush top-top secret. I was waiting outside to start filming a scene. There were strict rules about security. We were not allowed to take photographs and we were not allowed to tell anyone anything about the series. But someone else must have been wearing a spy camera, or maybe there were some paparazzi behind a hedge with long lenses on their cameras, because the next day there were photos of me on set and in my costume, standing next to my mum and the makeup people, waiting to film.

It was quite an interesting and worrying insight into how really famous people must live. Those photos started appearing in the *Daily Mail* and then the *Daily Express* and the *Sun*. Your name was in the top line. In fact, you were all over the press and during the day more and more photos of you kept on arriving in the online editions. Perhaps you were hot news at the time as you had just been on *Line of Duty* in that very emotive role. The stories went on for pages online and hardly mentioned the other, more famous actors.

It was really embarrassing. We had kept everything secret, but we worried that the film company would think we had leaked the photos. Would the company blame us? We needed people to be able to trust us to keep these secrets, or they might choose not to work with us again.

We phoned Rachael Swanston, your acting agent at Conway Van Gelder Grant, for advice. She checked with the production company who, to our relief, were understanding. They said we could mention you were in the film, but should not say anything about your character or the story. At least it was clear that I hadn't taken the photos, as they could see me in some of the longer shots, standing with you while you were waiting to film the scene.

It reminded me of when you were in *Line of Duty* and the phone kept pinging with all the lovely tweets coming in for you. Suddenly, incredibly, just overnight you had thousands of new followers on social media and so many kind comments about your performance.

I was pleased and proud to see all the messages from everyone. Thank you for supporting me. It really does mean a lot.

Chapter 17

Dance: feeling alive and free

Alongside acting, I truly love dancing. To me, dancing
means feeling alive and free to feel my emotions.
When I start dancing I really am the music. It just
flows through me and I can't help but move.

I remember watching you dance for Blue Apple and you
looked so happy. I thought to myself, we have to find more
dance for you.

One day, while I was still with Blue Apple, I was
being interviewed by Victoria Derbyshire with Sarah
Gordy MBE, who is also an actor who has Down
syndrome, and we talked about dance. Sarah told me
about her choreographer, Daniel Vais, the brilliant
artistic director of Culture Device who would later

create the production of *Waiting for Godot* that I enjoyed acting in so much. Daniel arranges live dance performances where he puts on music that fits what a person is suited to, and you improvise in front of the audience. He calls this post-contemporary dance. Improvising is one of my specialities. It can be really good fun to be a part of. I also reckon other people should start to improvise because it is one way of getting involved in dancing, and is also good for a warm-up exercise before you start.

I went for an audition with Daniel. He put on some music and just let me dance. He seemed to enjoy my stillness. Mum thought I wasn't doing enough, but Daniel could see what I was doing and that I was inside the music, or actually that I became the music. The one note he gave me was to use my back and shoulders more.

We've now done lots of projects together. Over the last ten years or so we've become great friends. Daniel is a true champion of artists with Down syndrome. He calls me 'Sir Tommy Jessop'!

When I'm working with Daniel, I might try improvising something in the warm-up session and then take it into the actual performance. We have performed our pieces at Somerset House, the Hackney Showroom, various art galleries and all over London. I also did a flashmob outside the Festival Hall on the South Bank in London about four years ago, which was fun. First I performed on stage with Daniel, and then I did some voguing with my dad as part of the flashmob. That was another thing Daniel had set up. It was enjoyable, but quite hilarious at the same time. I think my dad enjoyed doing it, and it is now part of our fitness regime. Dad likes teasing me about it. I don't think he had ever expected to perform in public outside the Festival Hall. I reckon he's a secret performer at heart, but doesn't really show it. I do enjoy watching him, it is quite entertaining.

In 2019, just before Covid, Daniel arranged for us to dance *The Rite of Spring* at the Royal Opera House in Covent Garden with other people with Down syndrome and members of the Royal Ballet. At first I did not know what to make of learning ballet, but eventually I grew into it. There is a lot about poise, posture and balance. The music for *The Rite of Spring* is by Stravinsky. It is edgy and wild, with quite a bit of tension and sudden energy. I do tend to thrive with dramatic music.

We had six weeks of rehearsing one day a week then a public performance with white costumes and a professional photographer. My whole family came to watch and so did lots of other people, including Sally Phillips and a few famous dancers.

Later, Daniel told me that he had been able to arrange this because the director had come to a Culture Device performance and been impressed by our dancing and interpretation of the music, and by our core strength.

Daniel really is doing a good job at arranging events for people with Down syndrome. I've already told you about *Waiting for Godot* in 2018, and more recently he invited me to dance in a programme he was planning for the Summer Festival at Somerset House in London. This was in August 2022. I was really looking forward to dancing with Sarah Gordy. I hadn't seen her since the December before, or danced with her in a long while.

I got my costume sorted out as well. I decided to go for all black because black is my favourite colour, and with my dance I want to create stillness and a thoughtful mood. I do enjoy making people think. I think the colour black makes people thoughtful and quite emotional as well.

The weather forecast for the day was 27 Celsius, which was steaming hot. There are some advantages and some disadvantages to having a heatwave. One advantage is having ice creams and banana milk shakes and smoothies. You get plenty of sunshine, which makes everything bright. The disadvantage of having a heatwave is that it is bad for the planet, because the warmer it gets the worse it is going to be for melting the glaciers and ice caps. You should have sun cream on at all times, wear shades and a hat as well. It is possibly wise to stay indoors between the hours of 12 noon and 4 p.m. because you might get skin cancer. A tour guide in Egypt told me that and it is sound advice. It is sound advice for the UK now too.

The event was called *This Bright Land*, and was hosted by Somerset House and Drag Syndrome, which is a collective of drag artists with Down syndrome. They were inviting other people too, like me. I was just dancing. I knew that when the time came and Daniel put the music on I would literally become the music itself.

It was an exciting and excitable day at Somerset House. Exciting because I was looking forward to performing, and excitable because the people watching seemed to enjoy my performance. I do enjoy people watching for the fun of it.

When we walked into the courtyard we could see a ferris wheel, a big stage and a catwalk. They had made little gardens round the side of the courtyard where you could sit under golden trees.

It had been a long while since I last saw Daniel Vais, so we had a quick chat about what he might be up to next. It was already hot, and one of the dancers almost fainted from the heat and after looking at the sun, which you should never do.

We met my dance partner Sarah Gordy in the green room. I hadn't seen her since we danced *The Rite of Spring* at Covent Garden before the curse of Covid cancelled everything.

There were five dances in total. I danced the first two as solos, then me and Sarah Gordy danced a duet, and Sarah did the last two solos. Then suddenly Daniel asked us to make speeches. I made a speech first, then it was Sarah's turn. Both of us were full of praise for Daniel for making everything happen, and I said that dance can make you healthy and strong.

How did you cope with it being so hot that day? The sun was burning through me while I was watching, and I was sitting still. You were dancing on stage and on the walkway in the sun. It must have been well into the mid–30s Celsius.

I must have felt so alive being able to express my emotions through the love and passion of music that I don't think I really noticed the heat. I did feel it a bit, but not much because I was lost in the music and dancing. I did feel a bit sweaty at the end of it, though. I had a can of ice-cold Sprite to cool down afterwards, which was refreshing.

At least there was a breeze to cool us a little as we walked back over the Thames to the station. It had been a great day. At the end of the bridge you can slip down into the food market by the South Bank Centre. I was looking for *arancini* to take home as a treat for supper. They had just sold out, but Tommy spotted a woman sitting on the steps with what looked like wonderful chips. We found the chips – they were cooked in duck fat and were about the best chips we had ever eaten. I don't know why we were so hungry in that heat, and I felt slightly guilty eating them. Dad was cooking supper for us. We were especially looking forward to this as your brother was coming round to join us for the meal in the garden. He is often so busy making films that we hardly ever see him. Ironically, when he's home you are often away!

Chips are one of the nation's favourite meals, and those duck fat chips were some of the best. I did not expect you to give some of those chips to a homeless person. It felt nice to give them some food. I felt warm inside at that time.

How do you feel when people watch you as you walk past? Three Chinese women with unusual tattoos asked for a selfie just as we were leaving Somerset House.

It was intriguing when they came up. I rather enjoy having selfies taken with people. It's wicked, because it means they have enjoyed my shows and being part of the occasion as well. That same week, Dad and I went to the supermarket because he was making pizzas and we needed mozzarella and tomatoes.

(His pizzas are pretty wicked. He makes them from scratch.) A woman came up in the check-out queue and asked for a selfie with me for her sister, who is twenty-two and has Down syndrome. She said I was an inspiration, which was reassuring. Another person in the queue asked what was going on, and mentioned that she had not watched *Line of Duty*. She might watch it on iPlayer now. There is a box set out too.

Anyway, on the way home from London our train was cancelled and while we were waiting we ate the duck fat chips, so waiting wasn't so bad. We caught the next train, and it was really cool in our carriage. I did some research on my phone, and a wordsearch puzzle as well.

It was quite crowded and there were lots of little children near us. One of the mothers said to them 'Relax your back and think happy thoughts.' It was one way to calm the children down. It worked. I will remember that.

Another thing I did with Daniel was to speak at the global launch of the Radical Beauty Project in

November 2022. Daniel believes that people with Down syndrome are full of radical beauty, and he loves contemporary art. I think that is why I like him so much, really. Starting in 2017, he found top photographers worldwide to take portrait photos of people with Down syndrome showing how beautiful they really are. The way the photographers do their photos is to put people in costumes, radical makeup and even masks. The photos taken of me changed my face in a different way. One photographer elongated it, and in the other photoshoot I was wearing a mask, which is quite funny really when the book is about showing how beautiful and gorgeous we really are! The mask was the gorgeous bit.

Daniel asked me to open the global launch event in London with a dramatic speech. As he wanted me to be theatrical, I wore my Hamlet jacket, which was fun.

In your speech you said 'We have an extra chromosome.' Then you paused, looked people in the eye, smiled and said 'It is a gift.'

People loved that. The room erupted with applause.

The launch was in a very large space, and Daniel projected our photos behind the stage. They were about ten feet high, with more around the room which were about four feet high.

I remember feeling how good it was that your voices were being heard and the thrill of being at an event where everyone was celebrating people with Down syndrome. All sorts of people were there from the arts and media worlds and a lot more photographs were taken. I remember you making your way round the room meeting everyone and catching up with old friends from Daniel's pre-Covid dance productions like *The Rite of Spring* with the dancers from the Royal Ballet at Covent Garden.

The best thing about the whole evening was that you could all simply be yourselves, some teasing each other, some serious, but all having fun. Everyone was there to celebrate your lives and, as Daniel would say, your beauty and your genius.

Chapter 18

Man on a mission

I love being an actor and an activist. Acting is my greatest passion and it makes me feel even more alive, but I've learned how important it is to speak up. I hope in my work I have helped other people to speak up for what they want to do in their lives.

Coming Down the Mountain, my first film in 2007, was all about making choices and knowing what you want out of life. My character, Ben, knew what he wanted, and had a girlfriend his family knew nothing about. He helped his older brother, David, to understand what he wanted out of his life too. Even my first play, *Adam*, in 2004, showed that my character had a gift and wanted to make his own decisions about his life. As I mentioned earlier, he wanted to be a chef and it turned out that, although no one believed him at first, he was a good chef.

I feel inspired by Dwayne Johnson, The Rock. He's known as The People's Champion by his wrestling fans. He is a voice for millions of people. I'd like to be a voice for people too.

So it might not be surprising to hear that one highlight in my life is being an activist. It is my acting that has given me a platform to speak out about issues I care about. In 2021 I joined the campaign for the new Down Syndrome Bill, campaigning for it to become law. This was a Private Members' Bill sponsored by Dr Liam Fox MP. It was introduced to the House of Lords by Baroness Hollins and supported by the National Down Syndrome Policy Group, whose members include several people with Down syndrome and health professionals. I was honoured and proud to become one of their Ambassadors.

This is the most important campaign that I have been part of because for too long people ignored our gifts and hid us away. We didn't learn anything and did not have jobs or get married. The Down Syndrome

Act is to make sure everyone with Down syndrome gets a proper education, with teachers understanding how we learn, better healthcare and real employment opportunities. For example, diagnostic overshadowing is an issue for us. It leads to healthcare professionals getting things wrong because they don't look at our symptoms properly. That really does scar us for life and can even kill us. I will tell you more about that later.

At the beginning of the campaign, I sent this email to MPs:

> Please will you support the Down Syndrome Bill?
>
> We need help from you by tomorrow if you can.
>
> Because it really is important for people to fulfil their lives and to be fulfilled.
>
> It is now time to improve and to celebrate people's lives worldwide.

What we really need is for people to believe in us and to understand us.

We all have skills, talents and gifts. We just need people to dig them out and those people also need to learn from us as well actually.

Thank you

From Tommy

Just before the first vote in the House of Commons, Tommy was invited to film a video message about the importance of the Down Syndrome Bill to him and to everyone, as he describes it, living with Down syndrome. This went to every single Member of Parliament before the second reading of the Bill. We were in semi-lockdown mode so, on 11 November 2021, I filmed him in the garden on my mobile phone with him mostly speaking to camera. It was a short piece but I think it had an effect and, certainly, in the end the Bill passed unopposed in both Houses of Parliament.

This is what I said in the video:

The most important thing for people with Down syndrome is to have a voice to speak up for what they really want in life and to show what they are truly capable of.

Don't tell us what to do, but help us make our own choices and live our everyday lives to the full.

I've been lucky, I've had brilliant support in my life.

I have a voice and I want to use it to help improve the lives of my friends and others who have Down syndrome.

Don't label us saying we can't do things. That's depressing and scars us for life. We can do things.

Everyone needs a bit of help from time to time.

It's time now for people with Down syndrome to have the same chances in life as anyone else.

We have waited long enough to be treated equally.

One day, 26 November 2021, just before the second reading in the House of Commons, I spoke outside Parliament to promote the Down Syndrome Bill.

That was a busy day actually. We started with a photoshoot for the *Guardian* quite early in the morning. Then we caught the train to London and walked across Westminster Bridge towards the Houses of Parliament with a documentary crew. It was quite windy. Mum wanted to stop and look at Big Ben, which had been repainted with a lot of gold and was sparkling in the sunshine. When we got to Parliament Square the place was full of people with Down syndrome and their families. I had a catch-up with Heidi Thomas, who as I mentioned had a brother with Down syndrome, and her husband Stephen McGann, who plays a doctor in *Call the Midwife*. I also caught up with another Heidi – Heidi Crowter, who is a brilliant campaigner who has Down syndrome. She keeps on going with her campaigning like a 'Duracell bunny'. She never gives up. Heidi can be hilarious, but there is something else impressive about her. She can be a diary of birthdays. She always knows who else has a birthday on your birthday. That is something me and Heidi have in common. We do tend to check out when other people's birthdays are coming up.

Lots of people from the media were there interviewing us, which was fun. I had a chat with people from the *Sun*, the *Daily Telegraph* and the BBC, and then did a live TV interview on the grass outside Parliament for ITV News. That morning I had also been on BBC Radio 4's *Today* programme giving out the same message, although that was a pre-record as I could not get into the studio to be live on air.

I enjoyed doing all that media, talking about how the lives of people with Down syndrome should be celebrated and could be improved by the Down Syndrome Act.

There are a couple more personal highlights from this campaign, like going to Number 10 Downing Street and standing on the doorstep, and also giving a speech at a reception in Parliament in March 2022, just before the third reading of the Down Syndrome Bill. Other people including Liam Fox, Baroness Hollins, Fionn Crombie Angus, who has Down syndrome, Gillian Keegan MP and Ken Ross from the National Down Syndrome Policy Group also made speeches. Being part of this made me feel really proud and honoured. You can read my speech here.

TO BE, OR...NOT TO BE?

My Lords, ladies and gentlemen, lend me your ears!

It really is a great honour to be here inside the House of Lords.

How brilliant.

We have a voice.

People are listening.

We have things to say.

So, to people with Down syndrome, I want to say: we are not all the same, we have different gifts,

believe in yourselves, be *kind*, and most of all, be who *you* want TO BE.

I watched Tommy lean his arm on the lectern and wait as cheering and applause echoed round the pavilion in the Palace of Westminster. He hadn't finished. He still had his final punchline to deliver. He took his time.

> So, I've thought about it, and I think it's better TO BE.
>
> Let's make history.

I like holding the room a bit too much. I do tend to enjoy being the centre of attention, and I feel comfortable making speeches. I'm getting used to public speaking. This was an important moment. We were celebrating. The Down Syndrome Bill was near to becoming law. I was proud and honoured to be a spokesperson for the Bill.

We had worked hard making speeches and giving interviews about how important the Bill was to us because it could change our lives. People with Down syndrome from all over the country had gathered at

Parliament and spoken out, and now the Bill is an Act. It will hopefully help professionals understand us better, and should celebrate our lives and improve our lives as well, through better healthcare, education, employment opportunities and housing.

Actually, Tommy, you are right. There really is a great need to share knowledge both about the way people with Down syndrome learn and about their health profiles, which can vary as much as within any other group of people. The Down Syndrome Act is important because too often medical diagnosis and teaching in school are overshadowed by the diagnosis of Down syndrome, with medical professionals attributing everything to the syndrome and not looking at the person properly or at their symptoms, and many teachers not expecting them to achieve much and not realising the person's potential. Parliament agreed that things need to improve and passed the Down Syndrome Bill.

There is a lot of valuable, practical and helpful research from people like Professor Sue Buckley, Director of Science and Research, Down Syndrome Education International, into how people with Down syndrome learn. Indeed, when running Blue Apple Theatre I was fascinated by the capacity and talents of our actors and dancers with

Down syndrome and am convinced that there is huge undiscovered potential amongst these lovely gentle people.

Hopefully the Act will identify, and incorporate into the training of healthcare professionals, teachers, social workers, housing executives and employers, the specific recognisable ways of helping people who have Down syndrome to live fulfilled, healthy and happy lives, discovering their gifts, becoming fully part of their local communities and reaching their potential as fully rounded human beings.

I would like to make even more speeches, sending out powerful messages to open other people's eyes to who we really can be, so that they listen to what people living with Down syndrome have to say. As I keep saying, that will happen if other people don't start by looking at the label, but instead look past it and really talk to the person himself or herself.

Tommy works hard on his speeches. Often he has new ideas when we least expect it, and quite often at mealtimes. He is mulling something over and then announces it. I tend to have a piece of paper nearby so that I can scribble these down! One of my favourites is 'Everyone has a gift. We just have to dig it out of them.'

Fact:

The Down Syndrome Act became law in April 2022. It is the first Act of its kind in the world.

Chapter 19

Changing our world
for the better

We can be proud and honoured that the Down Syndrome Bill has been passed and is now the Down Syndrome Act. It can also be history-making, changing the world for the better.

We really have waited long enough to be treated equally. It is time now for people living with Down syndrome to have the same chances in life that anyone else has, and not get hidden away.

Hopefully life will now improve. We will get proper care from people who believe in us, from teachers, doctors, nurses and employers too, just like everyone else, so we can all be healthy and happy and living our lives to the full.

That is what I have always done. I have been campaigning for better chances in life for people with Down syndrome all my acting career. I think others, including politicians, tend to label us, saying that we cannot do things. Except we can. People think we are all the same, but that is wrong too.

In summer 2022, we were invited to a party given by the US Embassy and Liam Fox to celebrate the passing of the Down Syndrome Act and I couldn't go! It was so tantalising. Tommy was to make a speech in front of VIPs and VVIPs at Winfield House, the American Ambassador's private residence near Regent's Park. It was a wonderful event.

He was only allowed ninety seconds which, with the way Tommy times and delivers his speeches, is just over a hundred words. So every word had to count. Fortunately Tommy had come up with some telling phrases over the previous few months.

I took quite few people to the embassy party, including a film crew I was working with at the time. Imogen Wynell-Mayow, the director of the *Panorama* documentary I was making, which I will tell you more about later, filmed me. Victoria Noble, our producer, came too, as did my friend Chris Pearce. I first met Chris at SNAPS Thumbs Up youth club when I was thirteen.

I usually go with Tommy to events like this to make sure he is comfortable with the venue, the lectern, and briefed about who he is meeting and keeps safe travelling. This time I had to explain all this carefully to Chris, who is a lovely guy, very easy to be with and understands Tommy well. I knew he would see him safely home. I was 300 miles away, but thanks to Chris's phone I saw the speech the next day and, once again, Tommy looked to be in his element, surrounded by kind faces and supporters.

To the reception I wore my black trousers, my usual trusty comfy shoes which are brown, and a black T-shirt and jacket. We travelled up by train and car because I was also being filmed for the *Panorama* documentary.

When we arrived the American flag was flying in the garden. I was looking forward to it all at that point. It was a sunny evening and we had drinks on the terrace. I drank champagne and then sparkling elderflower after the first glass.

There were a lot of people there, including Ambassador Philip Reeker, then the US Chargé d'Affaires in London, Dr Liam Fox MP, Baroness Hollins and other people from the House of Commons and the House of Lords, my friend Ken Ross from the National Down Syndrome Policy Group and the press. Most importantly, there were lots of people with Down syndrome and their families because the party was for us and our own Act, which is the first in the world to specifically help us.

I met people with Down syndrome that I had never met before, too. They were really nice, and some had come a long way to be there.

Ambassador Reeker, Ken Ross, Liam Fox and I all made speeches. I enjoyed making mine. I spoke about how the Act meant that we had made history. I said people with Down syndrome finally have a voice and it is about time people start listening to us and talking to us, finding out what we think and want, asking what our hopes and dreams might be.

Now we can decide what we want to say, and say it loud and clear. I don't think everyone finds that easy though, actually.

I said I wanted people to realise that people with Down syndrome are not all the same.

My big message was don't judge a book by its cover. That means don't simply label and dismiss us. Look past the label and see the people we truly are, who we really can be, believe in us.

Help people like me discover our gifts, find our skills and talents and show what we can do. That will mean a great big adventure for us and for the world.

I ended the speech by saying: 'Let's go and change the world for people living with Down syndrome!'

What happened next in this campaign, after the Bill became an Act, was that I joined a group of people with Down syndrome to discuss the next stages. This was in December 2022. The group is chaired by Fionn Crombie Angus, who has Down syndrome. We started talking to civil servants on Zoom about what could happen next, what is important to us and what can be improved. There were quite a few of us on the Zoom calls, but we all took turns speaking and it was wicked. I think some people might not need to talk quite so much on Zoom, some like to talk more! So the moderator makes sure everyone can speak and be heard.

Yet another one of my personal highlights of campaigning was going inside Number 10 Downing Street to talk to a minister with ten other people with Down syndrome from the National Down Syndrome Advisory and Policy groups. I felt honoured and proud to be there. I can't say what we discussed, but the minister gave us plenty of time to ask our questions. She seemed to understand what we were asking. Let's hope that our visit will help her in her job even more when she is thinking about people with Down syndrome.

The Down Syndrome Act has given people who actually have Down syndrome a voice for the first time. I hope we will now hear what they themselves feel, rather than try to speak for them. The Down Syndrome Act was conceived by, lobbied for and promoted by the National Down Syndrome Policy Group. This organisation has people with Down syndrome at its heart – a third of its founding members have Down syndrome, and all the other members are either parents or siblings who also run charities providing services to support people with Down syndrome in education, health and employment. As part of the National Down Syndrome Policy Group and the National Down Syndrome Advisory Group, which meets regularly by Zoom, people with Down syndrome are actively taking part in the consultations about implementing the Act and are now speaking up for themselves on public platforms. There are some very excited people with Down syndrome who love this chance to change the world they live in. Tommy is one of them.

Once I was working when the Advisory Group met, so I had to record a question for the panel with the civil servants who are writing the guidance. My question was important to me. I asked them what they would do to make sure there were more real jobs on offer for people with Down syndrome. I needed them to know how important this is. We are all different, and we can do different jobs. Once I thought I had a job, but I found out it was just sorting out coathangers. That is not a job.

Other real jobs that I have had include working in the MVC music store, as I mentioned previously. The manager, Jeremy, gave me the job of sorting out the CDs in the Top Ten and filling gaps on the shelves, which I quite enjoyed doing. I also enjoyed working in several libraries, including at Totton College, at my local hospital library and Winchester Library. That was fun. I was sorting out the library books into sections and then filling up the shelves in order. These could all be good jobs, but they were not what I dreamed about doing.

Now my job is being a professional actor, dancer and public speaker, and quite a bit of my TV work has been based in the NHS, actually: *Casualty*, *Holby City*, *Monroe*, *Panorama*, *Doctors*. Doctor, Doctor, I wonder why that is?!

I also do social media for a local charity and sometimes volunteer as an usher in the theatre, which I enjoy because I get to watch the shows for free, have ice creams in the interval and meet people while showing them to their seats.

I know people with Down syndrome with all sorts of jobs: someone who works in a library, someone who makes ice cream; a local councillor. I personally know models like Ellie Goldstein, actors like Sarah Gordy, Liam Bairstow, Leon Harrop and James Martin, whose short film won an Oscar, dancers like all of us at the Culture Device Dance Project, waitresses, TV presenter George Webster on CBeebies, drag queens like Justin Bond at Drag Syndrome, and other public speakers like me including Fionn Crombie Angus, who has spoken at the United Nations. I know a few competitive swimmers like Florence Garrett, gymnasts like Holly Riseborough, and a tennis player, Ben Tyler, who all represent Britain and compete in the Special Olympics. I know of a professional photographer, Oliver Hellowell, and a talented fashion designer, Isabella Springmuhl. I have even come across the very first female Zumba instructor, Hannah Payton, who has Down syndrome. Long may all this continue.

One exciting thing was being featured in the *Guardian* with other actors and models who have Down syndrome like Ellie, George and Zack Gottsagen. People are seeing us now.

People living with Down syndrome are diverse too, and we need to show this.

In 2022, Mencap asked me to become one of their Ambassadors. It made me feel really proud and it is an honour. Mencap is a charity that is passionate about changing the world for everyone with a learning disability. There are millions of people in the UK with learning disabilities, and I want to help Mencap make sure they can live their lives to the full and be happy and healthy. I hope to stop people saying that we can't do certain things. Instead people should all be saying 'Yes, you can.'

I enjoyed going to Mencap's Carols by Candlelight service that Christmas and reading for them in St Bartholomew the Great, in Smithfield, London. The church is one of the oldest in London, and it has been used as a location for films like *Four Weddings and a Funeral* and *Shakespeare in Love*. I chose my own reading. It was a few lines from 'Christmas' by John Betjeman, about the most tremendous tale of all.

I had a good chat and a laugh with Johnny Ball after the service, and with other people from Mencap. Johnny Ball used to present science and maths on children's television and writes fun maths books for children. He is still mad keen on maths. Johnny was also reading. His piece was 'Twas the Night Before Christmas'. He does have a really good reading voice.

*   *   *

Another very important thing that I have been campaigning for is much better healthcare for people with learning disabilities. I am on a mission to see what can be done to improve this.

So, in 2022 I made a documentary for *Panorama* about this. I met people around the country to see what their experience of accessing healthcare had been. That documentary came out in October that year, and it's something I've taken the most pride in doing in my campaigning career so far. I will tell you more about what it was like later.

I also felt proud and honoured when I found out that someone had nominated me for the 2022 Shaw Trust Disability Power 100 List. I was in the entertainment section with Rose Ayling-Ellis, who won *Strictly Come Dancing* and changed the lives of people who are deaf. It was truly wicked that people voted for me.

The next thing in my campaigning career was the Southampton City of Culture Bid for 2025. They asked me to become one of their Ambassadors. I agreed so long as they included in the bid plans for providing real cultural opportunities for people with learning disabilities to take part in theatre, music, dance and so on, not just as audience members in relaxed performances. Sadly, we didn't win the bid, but I hope it's a start for all kinds of culture to come together as one big family.

I was also asked to become Patron of the Portsmouth Down Syndrome Association, who campaign and run lots of projects for people with Down syndrome. As part of that we had dinner on HMS *Warrior*. I sat with rugby players, who were talking about their rugby injuries and sang sea shanties. Another event was a garden party where I had to meet lots of people and talk to them. There I met a stunt double who had worked on a James Bond film. I told him I wouldn't mind playing James Bond one day!

My work as a campaigner and as an actor gives me lots of different ways to help change minds and be a spokesperson for people with Down syndrome. I'm always ready for the next challenge.

Chapter 20

Talking sport

You may have found out by now that I love sport. It's my favourite topic of conversation. One of my many hobbies in life is football. My favourite thing about watching or playing football is the feeling of enjoyment when we score a goal and the crowd erupts in cheering. Kicking a football and the feel of the ball on my foot is wicked.

My ambition for my team is winning the Premier League, and to get into the Champions League as well. This might even come true. If things continue to go as well as they are while I'm writing this book, we might be in the Champions League for the first time in nearly twenty years. Let us hope they carry on winning!

Well, when my team wins a Premier League game, let's just say that earplugs are needed for my next-door neighbours. And when my team loses a Premier League game I tend to go quiet, which is not a pleasant sight apparently.

I am really excited about supporting Newcastle United because they are now the richest Premier League team. I do find it intriguing and exciting trying to find out who we get to play for us next. I am actually glued to the transfer news. The latest players we have brought in include Alexander Isak from Sweden, Kieren Trippier, who is English, and Nick Pope, who is a brilliant goalkeeper, one of the best we have had. I think we have even built our best defence this season.

On my past holidays, I have asked many people what football teams they support. I reckon that football is all about teamwork and helping other people out when they need it most. It is a game being played worldwide, and is known as the Beautiful Game. And it might also be a way of getting to know people and making new friends anywhere around the world. I've talked about football in Namibia, which was one place I enjoyed visiting, and also Egypt. In Morocco I asked my killer question when I was dancing with the winner of the belly-dancing competition. She saw me dancing and came over and asked me to dance with her. She said her prize for winning the competition was to dance with me!

The people I ask about their favourite football team usually used to support Manchester United, but now it is Arsenal. I might be on a mission to find out if there are any Geordie supporters around – that basically means Newcastle United fans. In the next country I visit, I will find out.

In Namibia I met the Ju|'hoansi San Bushmen of the Kalahari and talked about football with Freddie, who was our guide when we went hunting and gathering in the desert. We didn't just talk about football, though. We also talked about life as a bushman, and about seeds and roots and porcupines and elephants. But football helped when it was so hot that I got tired and had to have a sit-down rest with them.

Over twenty-six years ago I watched my very first Premier League game live and in person, and it really was an enjoyable afternoon trip. Newcastle were playing Southampton at home. So I had to go all the way to Newcastle to their old stadium, but I had to sit in the Saints seats because it was so difficult to get tickets. I think Matt Le Tissier was playing then. He scored the winning goal for Southampton and I had to keep my mouth shut. I reckon that particular game really did scar me for life!

How the mighty have fallen and the underdogs have risen since then. I was a bit nervous before I went to a match recently with my brother because we had to sit in the Saints area again as all the Newcastle seats were sold. I did not wear my Newcastle United shirt as it might have sparked controversy!

But for this match I really did enjoy sitting with the Saints fans. I knew we were going to beat them. In the past the Saints away team always tended to win, and this game was at their home ground. So up north Saints might have beaten us, but down south we beat them. I think we might also be a curse against Saints because we do seem to get rid of their managers.

After this particular game their manager was given the sack, sadly.

We had to walk a mile and a half through the rain to get to the stadium. The streets were full of fans walking with us. Most people were in coats to keep off the rain. Most of the Saints fans were quiet and the most raucous fans were the Geordies, perhaps because they felt confident we were going to win. I was looking forward to the match, looking forward to a win, but I felt nervousness with a hint of excitement.

I really enjoyed watching it. I was on the edge of my seat, quite literally. We were not expecting Saints to score against us, but they had about sixteen shots on target and all but one were saved by our brilliant goalie, Nick Pope. Nick Pope and Chris Wood and Kieran Trippier all used to play for Burnley together so they know each other well. I thought that Kieran Trippier would definitely play in the World Cup, which was coming up two weeks later, because he really is good at influencing games. In our game he was feeding Miguel Almirón, who scored the first goal. He plays for Paraguay and he had been with Newcastle for about a year. When Almirón scored, I was sitting in the Southampton seats and we had a rule about not celebrating, but inside I was. I just clenched my fists and enjoyed the cheering from the Newcastle seats.

Football matches can be quite loud. When I was younger they were too loud, but this time I enjoyed the chants that were coming from the Geordies, including 'When the mags go marching in'. When the next goals were scored there were two former Arsenal players on the pitch, which really was intriguing to watch, along with the three former Burnley players playing for us. One of them is really good at scoring from free kicks. We also have really good players from Brazil, actually.

Talking about football, my friend Ben had a birthday on the day of a big World Cup match. It was England against world champions France. His family turned the sofas round so that we could all watch their TV and we started with champagne. Then it was the kick-off. It was painful to watch because France truly are the world champions. I actually reckon they really were lucky to win. But on the other hand I really did enjoy myself being there. I had a delicious supper, and they have a really nice dog called Pippa. She really is very cute, and the kind of dog that I like, a very silent one.

Interesting football facts:

- The FA Cup is the oldest national football competition in the world. It started in 1871.

- The Premier League was only founded in 1992.

- The Champions League started in 1955.

- The offside rule was introduced in 1883. The basic rule is that you can't pass the ball forward to a player on your team unless there are at least two players from the defending team between them and the goal, but there are a lot of complications.

On the subject of sport, I'm also a tennis fan. My favourite player is Rafa Nadal, because I like the style he plays with. He never gives up, no matter how he is playing or how the match is going. I like the philosophy he carries around with him. He tends to be really caring, strong-minded and focused, a brilliant tennis player. My second-favourite tennis player is none other than Cameron Norrie, for a very good reason. I found out that he supports Newcastle United. I wanted Cameron Norrie to win last year's Wimbledon in honour of Rafa Nadal after he was injured. That was a real shame as I had hoped Rafa was going to win all four Grand Slams in the calendar year.

Rafa Nadal does not know when he might be beaten, so he always puts up a really good fight. He is a game changer when he turns matches round to win. To me, Rafa is now the GOAT – which means the Greatest Of All Time – in the world of tennis players, which makes me pleased for him. When he loses a game I do not react at all well, and I want the player who has beaten Rafa to lose his next match, just to feel the same pain Rafa is going through for losing. I care because I really do not like seeing Rafa in pain through defeat or through injury.

In fact, I do not like anyone to be in pain. I feel their pain as well, because I can fully relate to them. This is why I can be an agony uncle. If any of my friends are in pain they can always come to me to put them in a really good mood. I am be there to be good company and cheer people up. I think I can quite easily share these painful feelings against the world. They say a burden shared is a burden halved. I like that phrase.

I have some tennis facts too:

- The Wimbledon Tennis Tournament was first held in 1877, but it was just for male tennis players. The women's championships began in 1884.

- In the nineteenth century, women played in long white dresses and hats and men had to wear long trousers. They must all have been pretty hot.

- Tennis seems to have started from a medieval French handball game, *jeu de paume*. It was like tennis but played without rackets, so it was called 'game of the hand'. The Jeu de Paume in Paris has become an art gallery.

Chapter 21

Singing my heart out

You already know how much I love music and dancing (as well as football). My other great passion in life is actually singing. I love singing my heart out.

I feel proud and quite emotional when I start singing, because I can encourage other people to start singing too. I reckon singing is really important, because it's something you can do whenever you want, no matter how happy or sad you are. You can just be yourself, and be free to sing about your emotions to the world.

Singing with other people really does help as well, actually. Another of my other mottos is that communication is key in life, and singing helps you to communicate.

I sing every week. My singing group has been going for four whole years and we've made up our own songs as well as singing 'When the Saints Go Marching In', 'Swing Low Sweet Chariot', 'Electricity', 'Rolling in My Sweet Baby's Arms', 'Teenage Dirt Bag', 'Hakuna Matata' and 'Shake It Off' by Taylor Swift.

Our own songs are called 'Here We Stand' and 'Don't Worry, Be Happy'. We made them up ourselves, which is wicked, so they are Blue Apple originals. I do like making up songs in our singing group.

The very first performance that we did was at the Railway Inn in Winchester. We have also performed in Eastleigh, Basingstoke and the Winchester Hat Fair on numerous occasions. I enjoyed all the performances and the rehearsals. Singing to an audience means you can share the love of music.

Last December, the singing group did a performance at the Winchester Christmas Market. We put on our Christmas hats and sang about four of our favourite songs and three Christmas songs. It really was fun to do. I wore my Santa Claus falling down the chimney hat. The hat itself is the chimney and Santa is on top, falling down it. I do tend to wear this at Crimbo time every year.

The songs that we sang were 'Baby It's Cold Outside', 'Half the World Away', 'Put a Little Love in Your Heart', 'Jingle Bells', 'We Wish You a Merry Christmas' and 'The Twelve Days of Christmas'. We did some warm-ups on stage as it was so cold. It was about minus one. When we sang our breath became warm and steamy in the cold air, like dragons' breath. People gathered round and some children started dancing just in front of the stage. I enjoyed watching them dancing. Sometimes I can't help dancing while we are singing.

After the performance I had a Bratwurst with curry sauce on it from one of the stalls at the Christmas Market for my tea, which really was nice.

Last summer we also sang at the Winchester Hat Fair, which was wicked to be a part of. Being the centre of attention was fun and I enjoyed having a laugh with other people. We sang 'Hakuna Matata', and I used sign language to help get the audience singing and laughing with us. Then we sang our own song, 'Don't Worry, Be Happy', and the audience joined in again.

Soon after that, we went to the last singing group of the summer term. It was also the last singing session for Kate Mellors, who was running it, as she was leaving. I feel emotional about that because she's quite irreplaceable. She's taught us timing and composition and singing in tune and she makes everyone feel happy. She's taught us extremely well.

Thankfully the singing group is still going on and the new singing leader is called Nicola Dunscombe. She is doing a really good job in taking over the reins from Kate. I think our singing is getting better. We are currently singing Bon Jovi's 'Living on a Prayer', Sam Ryder's 'Spaceman', 'You are the Music in Me' from *High School Musical* and Toto's 'Africa'.

I used to think that opera really wasn't my thing at all. But there was a saying in my mind at that time, which was 'It isn't over until the fat lady sings.' Except she usually starts singing at the very start, apparently. I saw *Tosca* at the Theatre Royal when I was working there, and then in New York with Will and my mum when we were at the Emmy Awards. I've also seen *The Yeomen of the Guard* at the Grange Festival. *The Yeomen of the Guard* was a bit like Hamlet, my favourite Shakespeare play, but there is a gunshot, whereas Hamlet has a sword. There is a case of mistaken identity and some romance as well. My favourite character was the court jester, actually. Seeing these productions has changed my mind about opera. I enjoyed them and might enjoy opera even more having seen them.

It really is worth going to the opera, and I highly recommend people try it. I also recommend everyone sings in the shower.

Interesting facts about singing:

- No one really knows who invented music, but singing might be older than speaking and it might be the oldest organised sound.

- Sound comes out of our mouths at approximately 75 miles per hour.

- And another interesting fact: our voices are as unique as our fingerprints.

Chapter 22

In the media

There is yet another personal highlight in my career, and that is being in the media, and all of the publicity I get to do, both promoting my professional acting work and especially for my campaigning. I take great pride in doing press interviews like the *Guardian*'s 'Meet the Gamechangers' feature, and being interviewed on shows like *Good Morning Britain*, making a video for LADbible and recording podcasts.

This started with a lot of publicity in 2007 when *Coming Down the Mountain* was shown on BBC One. I think there were features about you in every national newspaper and many regional ones too, plus lots of radio and television interviews.

I like getting my own voice across in interviews, and it is fun going to photoshoots.

One of the features for the *Guardian* involved a photoshoot in July 2021 with photographer Sophia Spring and model Ellie Goldstein in a studio in London where everything was white. They had a whole rail of designer clothes for you to wear and you ended up with a lovely fluffy Paul Smith jumper in bright colours.

They also styled me in a Gucci jumper for some other shots. Ellie was quite a character to work with and I enjoyed choosing the clothes to wear. I would have chosen to keep some of them, but that wasn't an option!

You did some shots together with Ellie, leaning on a white block. They had invited a *Guardian* journalist to interview each of you. The journalist asked you all about your career, about filming *Line of Duty* and your dreams for the future. You told them 'Never judge a book by its cover.'

The feature was headlined 'Six Stars with Down's Syndrome Lighting up our Screens: People are talking about us instead of hiding us away. Meet the Gamechangers.' The front cover of the magazine featured Ellie, Australian model Madeline

Stuart, George Webster from CBeebies and US actors Zack Gottsagen and Kassie Mundhenk.

I do like the name 'Gamechangers'. The clue is in the title. Look where we are right now.

Sometimes a lot of media interviews can come at once. I do not mind this. I really do look forward to doing them. I mostly answer straight away, but I like taking a short time to think about what I want to say. That means pre-records are easier, because if it is live you might not always have enough time to think of your answers straight away.

I will just tell you about a busy few months around *Line of Duty* winning at the National Television Awards and campaigning for the Down Syndrome Bill.

In September 2021 I recorded a podcast for Spotlight, the actors' agency. I think that was all about being in *Line of Duty*. On 11 November 2021 I filmed my message to all MPs explaining why the Down Syndrome Bill was so important to us, and the next day I recorded a podcast about my life and being an

257

actor and why I felt the Down Syndrome Bill mattered so much.

Soon after, on 22 November, I did a pre-record for ITN News and the next day I recorded an interview with Martha Kearney for BBC Radio 4's *Today* programme. That afternoon I went into a recording studio to record a song for Blue Apple Theatre.

On 3 December 2021, I had a Zoom interview for the *Guardian* for their topic 'The Outspoken'. They wanted to write 2,000 words about me and about my campaigning, and this was followed by a photoshoot in January. That time I had to walk through a beautiful wood with photographer Victoria Adamson.

This was for a solo feature later in the year, which was prompted by your campaigning for the Down Syndrome Bill, and for greater understanding of the gifts and potential of people living with Down syndrome.

I enjoyed that photoshoot, like I do all of them, really. At some photoshoots they put on loud music so that you feel relaxed and in a good mood. They might style your hair and give you a choice of clothes to wear. Sometimes there are snacks.

As one of their Ambassadors, I did a photoshoot for Mencap in December 2021 that I really enjoyed. My friend Sarah Gordy was just finishing her session when I arrived, so we had a quick chat. We had not seen each other since before Covid, when we danced *The Rite of Spring* with members of the Royal Ballet and other dancers with Down syndrome at Covent Garden.

The photographer was India Whiley-Morton. She is Jo Whiley's daughter. Jo is also a Mencap Ambassador and was a DJ on BBC Radio 1 when I was younger, one of my favourite Radio 1 DJs. Now she is on BBC Radio 2. I did not know India was her daughter at the time, but we did have a good connection. We were in a big warehouse with white walls. Mencap were filming us while we did the shoot, so there were quite a few cameras around.

Mencap announced that I was their new Ambassador in January 2022, so I did several interviews then about why I agreed to become a Mencap Ambassador, about my life and acting and about the Down Syndrome Act. On 7 January I had Zoom interviews with the *Mirror* online and the *Daily Express*. On 10 January I had an interview with *OK!*

Magazine and on 11 January I was on *BBC Breakfast* and *Good Morning Britain*, the articles in the *Mirror* and *Express* appeared and I was also in *The List* and *Learning Disability Today*. The main reason why I had that many interviews was that they were planning to do them in one whole day, but I felt that was a bit too much. I prefer to do one interview at a time, so we planned to do them in a week instead.

On 15 January I think I might have taken Alastair Stewart by surprise. He interviewed me for *Alastair Stewart & Friends* on GB News in January 2022 about becoming an Ambassador for Mencap. The interview was live and went off really well, even though he changed the questions I thought he would ask me! He was joyful and thoughtful. We talked about people with learning disabilities not getting enough support to do interesting things like going to work, or to youth clubs, or getting good healthcare, and that being labelled separates us and makes us feel we can't do things.

One thing I said was that I wanted people to stop saying 'No, you can't' and say instead 'Yes, you can', and give us a chance to show who we really can be in life.

That was the day our football teams were playing against one another. So just at the end of the interview I surprised him with my killer question about what team he supported. That made Alastair laugh.

On 26 January I particularly enjoyed filming an interview with LADbible, who have done interviews with actors like Mark Wahlberg. I was in quite a dark studio with cameras and microphones all over the place, including one just over my head. I talked about jobs, schools and my career. We had spoken several times on Zoom beforehand so we were all well prepared and I felt very relaxed. This came out of being in *Line of Duty*.

I really did enjoy my photoshoot for my very own memoir in December 2022. You can see the photo they took on the jacket of this book. There might have been some dancing, with Alexa supplying the music, and there was really good company. Pål Hansen was behind the camera. He has taken photos of Nicole Kidman, Elton John, Mark Rylance, Bill Nighy, Graham Norton, Daniel Radcliffe and Ralph Fiennes, amongst others, who are all people I admire. That really is an all-star and impressive list.

There was really nice food for lunch as well, which Alex, my very own publisher, went out to get. Alexa kept on changing the music, which was wicked, and the room that we were in was very spacious. It had a ceramic hob and one of the people there made me a really nice hot chocolate.

Patrick, who designed the cover, and Pål chose the colours for the photoshoot, and I chose the clothes with the help of my stylist Andie Redman.

With the lovely clothes and the music I could not help dancing. I probably feel like that all of the time. Even without the music playing I actually do feel like dancing the whole time.

Ever since *Coming Down the Mountain* the media have been asking you about your life and work, and this continues, but those months were so incredible. And in between all this media you have been working, making public speeches and writing this book!

I enjoy doing the media interviews, but it can get quite tiring. It's good to get the questions in advance to think about, but who knows what other questions might come up. As I have mentioned, when I'm being interviewed I might ask my very own question, like what football team the interviewer supports, and find out what their favourite hobbies are. It is one way of finding out what they are like, though it takes the interviewer by surprise.

Since 2021, you have become Ambassador for Mencap, Ambassador for the National Down Syndrome Policy Group, an honorary Doctor of Arts at the University of Winchester, Ambassador for Southampton City of Culture 2025 and Patron of the Portsmouth Down Syndrome Association. Each of these organisations has given you a chance to speak about what is important to you and to other people with Down syndrome, and we have seen you grow so much in confidence that you are now booked as a public speaker, travelling to conferences around the country.

Now I have added a role as a journalist, finding out about other people's lives and trying to help them.

Chapter 23

My first investigation: *Panorama*

I have made documentaries before with my brother and acted in films about improving healthcare for people with learning disabilities. In 2022, I had the chance to film my own documentary for *Panorama* on BBC One: *Will the NHS Care For Me?* It was my first project as an investigative journalist. There were a few ups and downs and knocks and bruises along the way, but I enjoyed myself doing it.

It is quite a tough story, in fact. I was totally a man on a mission to find out what people with learning disabilities really are going through in hospitals, and to listen to what they have to say.

I'm hoping we can improve healthcare because some people with learning disabilities are dying too soon from things that could be prevented. People with learning disabilities are twice as likely to die from avoidable causes as other people. This does not seem fair. It is frightening. That is why I decided to make the film.

Immy – Imogen Wynell-Mayow – was the director of the new documentary. The first time we met Immy she mentioned that she can be a bit clumsy and gets lost easily, and that basically meant I had to show Immy all around town. One of the other names I have is 'Satnav'. That is literally true. I'm always showing and telling people where to go.

Victoria Noble was the producer, as I mentioned earlier. Immy brought Vicky down to meet us, to talk about the itinerary for the filming process and how it would pan out.

We were sitting outside at a café because of Covid, sheltering by the wall because it was so windy. It was still March, and pretty cold. We ordered hot chocolate, which arrived with cream on top, and someone got cream on their nose.

That is true. Vicky got cream on her nose! Hot chocolate is a reassuring drink to have to keep you energised and also help you relax a bit more. I like having hot chocolate in the morning for elevenses and at night time as well.

I enjoyed the food intake while we were on location for the documentary, especially pizza after a hardworking day, and most of all the good company of people that I was working with.

Once we had lunch at a steak house, and we also had fish and chips by the sea in Taunton. A man came up and asked what we were filming, but Immy would not tell him. Most of my TV and film work has to be top-secret, and I can understand why, but it can really be quite annoying not being able to tell people what I am doing in my career.

In Sheffield we did an interview with a learning disability nurse. She was friendly and fun, but her job was intense. I felt sorry for her having to cope with the pressure of her work. We agreed that the healthcare system should be better at understanding people with learning disabilities. She said there are not enough learning disability nurses to help doctors. Learning disability nurses understand how to communicate and look after a person who has got a learning disability. I reckon we all need learning disability nurses. We also met Dr Charley Annesley at North Middlesex University Hospital. We sat outside as it was a really hot day and there was still some Covid around. Dr Charley is a designated consultant who sees every adult patient with a learning disability who is admitted for whatever reason to make sure that nothing is overlooked. She was friendly and smiley and easy to talk to. I think we should have a Dr Charley in every hospital.

Next day we went to the Peak District to meet someone who had had a sad experience.

That story did need to be told.

We did a lot of the work in May 2022, when I met some families of people with learning disabilities who had died. It can be distressing and they are suffering with their loss, and I might be someone who can help to guide them through. That might mean listening to them remember all of the good things about their loved ones who they have lost, like how much a lovely person living with Down syndrome had enjoyed singing and dancing.

Afterwards Immy filmed you sitting on a bench in Sheffield.

At that point I really was fed up with the way the healthcare system was handled and how much it could be improved.

It seems that sometimes doctors assume a person's illness is part of their disability when it isn't, and also sometimes people don't value the life of a person who has a learning disability so they don't help them properly. This is very upsetting for them and for their families, and some people die.

My mum and I kept a diary of one of the weeks of making the documentary so that we can describe what it was like.

May

Vicky and Immy are delightful and fun, and very aware of how hard Tommy might find it being invited into people's homes and hearing their stories. It's Thursday and we are all trying to make sure he is OK. He listens well, and with sympathy. He seems fine. He seems able to keep things separate. We are trying not to dwell on the bad stories but, when we are travelling or eating together, to keep talking about his hobbies and interests.

Tommy is standing in the hot sun in Sheffield, his eyes beginning to close. He's been talking to these lovely people for a while now. They care so much about the young woman who died so suddenly in hospital. I think they have made him half fall in love with her with their talk of her kindness, her beauty, her love of singing and dancing. Now he has to thank them for talking to him. He goes quiet. We wait. It should be simple just to say a quick 'Thank you for talking to me.' We wait a little longer. There's a pause, he looks aside, thinking. Then his words come, 'This has been a painful story to hear, but it has to be told. Thank you.'

I had a mixture of feelings, anger and sadness.

I hope the stories do not go in too deep, and I don't want Tommy to be scared if he has to go into hospital in the future. At least we filmed a lovely interview with a GP this morning, demonstrating best practice in annual health checks.

On Friday I went to a solicitor's offices to learn more about coroners' reports, and this was where I got my war wound. I went to go through what I thought was the door, and I bumped my head on the curved glass panel that looked like a revolving door. On the other hand, one person who worked there actually did say that I was even more good-looking than Tom Cruise. I was lying down at the time with ice on my head, so watch out TC!

Frontlining this documentary has taken Tommy to some hard places, but that evening we go out for a pizza with the lovely Immy and then sleep at the Travelodge in Bethnal Green. Tommy had a relaxing time, laughing with Immy and enjoying the pizza and a chocolate ice cream.

That is the main documentary stunt work out of the way, actually. Now I can have a break while they do the edit.

It's Wednesday and I just had a Zoom meeting with Immy, Vicky and the production team. The BBC like the film so far, but Immy can't finish the edit yet. They're still researching a new story, and they might need to make changes. So it will not be shown until the autumn now.

On Friday, I will be doing a voiceover for the documentary to test out the sound and see how long we have for explaining things. Vicky is coming to our house with a microphone and the script and we'll work in our quietest room. I quite miss going up to London, but it is possibly wise doing this at home because there is a rail strike, and Covid as well. So I'll have a shower to get ready and warm up my vocal chords by having a good sing in that very shower. It should be wicked seeing Vicky. We might have a laugh as well.

When Vicky arrives we talk about the stories and try doing the voiceover three different ways to make it sound right. I have to sit very still so we don't make any noise.

Sometimes I sound really passionate about it all, because some of what we found out is bad. I do feel sorry for the all the families who might have lost people too soon and are going through a painful time. Hopefully our film will help improve the healthcare that people with learning disabilities are given.

We get a bit hungry doing all this, and Vicky's tummy is rumbling, which is not a good sound for a documentary, so we have some biscuits. It is thirsty work too, but I enjoy doing it. I feel it is really important to show everyone the need to improve healthcare for people with learning disabilities in the NHS.

Afterwards we have a good chat about football. I've got two pieces of intriguing information about football matches for Vicky and Immy, and about the football teams they support. In the Championship the fixtures have just been released. Derby County will be playing against the team where Immy grew up, Oxford. Our first game is Newcastle against Nottingham Forest, who are one of the newly promoted teams, and the third game will be against Vicky's team, West Ham. After that discussion, Vicky knew quite a bit about football, mostly through me. I reckon that she might turn into a Geordie. I'm working on her to support my team, and I hope that one day we might film in Newcastle so that we can go to the stadium together.

On Saturday I finish the last bit of filming with Immy. Afterwards we have lunch to celebrate all our work on the documentary.

It was hard work, but I reckon that people with learning disabilities of all kinds should be treated equally, fairly and respected in healthcare and everywhere else.

I am honoured and proud to have been invited into the homes and lives of people who have been through really hard and sad times. They have suffered.

The programme is called *Will the NHS Care for Me?* I reckon the NHS will care for us if we care for it. That means providing good training, staffing and money. It was broadcast in October 2022. I enjoyed doing the publicity for the programme. I also enjoyed watching it back at the screening that *Panorama* arranged at the BBC. We invited producers, families from the film and other influential people, and had an after-party after the screening, which was fun.

I made a speech about all the hard work put into the film, and about the families and how they should be heard. I hope we gave them a voice.

There was lots of publicity about the documentary, and Immy and I were interviewed for BBC Radio

4's *PM* programme too. She was quite nervous beforehand, but I was there to make sure she was OK. I enjoy doing interviews and getting a powerful message across.

So my main message is that these hard-hitting stories about the lives these people have been through really should be told. Then healthcare for people with learning disabilities will improve.

At least, I hope so!

Chapter 24

If you ask me

Perhaps it is time to tell you a bit more about me and my reflections on life and friendship. First I will tell you about things that make me happy, and then some things I find difficult.

I reckon that acting, dancing, listening to music, laughter, supporting football teams, friends, family and people saying 'Well done' make me feel happy. The trouble is that sometimes some of these things can also make you sad. Like football teams. I was happy my football team had not lost a Premier League game, but sad when they started going downhill again.

Being in character when I am acting and having a really good talk with the other actors and crew about films or sport or teasing each other between scenes makes me happy. When I'm on a film set it is like being a team member or a member of a family, and everyone works together to make the film a success. It's teamwork, being in a film. Everyone helps everyone else to do a good job. So being in a film is a happy place.

Researching on my iPad or my phone makes me feel happy. I like finding out certain news, such as football transfers, knowing whose birthdays are coming up and checking out film reviews. Getting a new script to read is always brilliant too. When I'm at home, I like walking to the shop to buy my magazines and calling in on my brother on the way home for a coffee. I also enjoy playing a game and listening to loud music with Dad. That is wicked, actually. He plays Creedence Clearwater, the Beatles and the Kinks, which makes Mum get up and dance in the kitchen. Some days we can't stop dancing. I love the sound of music, especially Dad's piano playing, and that of church singing, bacon sizzling, and Mum singing and laughing.

But I don't like the sound of fireworks, smoke alarms, ambulance sirens, babies crying, or dogs barking. This might be because they are sudden sounds. When a dog barks or runs towards me I do tend to avoid it at all costs. I am intrigued by how dogs think. I am worried not for their owners, but for other people walking past because dogs jump up and you can't get away. Their owners say they are just being friendly, but that doesn't help. I still dread them jumping up, because even if they are friendly they still might do it suddenly.

With fireworks, I look out of the window to see what they are. They are beautiful, but I prefer listening to them from inside the house. Outside the noise is a bit too loud. Some fireworks can make sudden noises which can make you jump. But one Saturday night I decided to face my fears and went to my second Bonfire Night in person with my brother, who was filming the whole thing. I enjoyed it, and the fireworks didn't all seem noisy, which is quite rare, and both surprising and pleasing. I don't mind other loud sounds, but sudden sounds can make me feel twitchy and fed up. I know when babies cry they can't help doing it, but it is quite annoying. Some people with Down syndrome take it personally when babies cry and think they are crying about them. But they are not. Babies might cry because they need food or a bit of tlc or a clean nappy.

Talking about things happening suddenly, I do tend not to react at all well when things happen at short notice. It is a case of getting my head round it all. I think sometimes it is the same for other people too. I understand about short notice – maybe a bit too much. It is all about timing and not making things happen too suddenly, which can be stressful.

My message about asking me to do things at short notice is always to tell my mum first. If you do that, it will give me a bit of a time to think things through and be comfortable. I might not reply straight away, but I will think about it quietly. Then I can be ready and on good form for what is needed. On a film set, we ask people to tell my mum about changes to timings and things so we can talk about it quietly and not in a rush. Then I am fine, even if I only have a couple of minutes to take the change on board. I like to have time to think about auditions too. That means I can look forward to them, enjoy getting into character and do the audition really well. However, short-notice auditions are better than no auditions!

My main message is to talk to me about what is happening. Then I can get my head round it. Other people probably feel the same way. Explain, then we can understand and get on with things.

Rushing is another thing that can put pressure on people. I know I do not react at all well to it. Rushing makes me feel a mixture of panic and feeling out of control, and I tend to go a bit too quiet. I do quite well when put under pressure, and I can be quick when I need to be – it is the last-minute rush or walking too fast, haring along, that is difficult. I need to take my time when walking, especially when there are steps. While some people can be a bit too quick, though, other people are a bit too slow for their own good. I know they can't really help it, but at the same time I wish they could walk a tiny bit faster. So I do understand what other people might feel like!

Facts about speed:

- England's fastest land animal is the brown hare, which runs at 43 miles per hour. That's why I said 'haring along' when I meant someone going very quickly.

- The fastest land animal in the world is the cheetah, which can run at 70 to 80 miles per hour for short distances.

- The peregrine falcon is even faster than a cheetah. It can fly at 242 miles per hour.

To the list of things I find hard I can add really tall buildings such as churches, cathedrals and skyscrapers, and talking to very tall people. These all make you look up, and I tend to freeze and shudder when I look up at certain things. That makes it difficult to look at tall people when I am talking to them, so they do not hear what I am saying, especially at parties. It appears that I might not be the only person with this phobia. I have a friend who shudders when he goes into a tall or big theatre space, and it is definitely reassuring that I am not the only one who feels like this.

I reckon that signposts should be put at a much lower height as well as high up, like they do for pedestrian crossing lights. Signs in hospitals and stations and signposts can be really high, and you can get lost quite easily if you cannot look up at them.

Facts about looking up:

- The International Space Station orbits the earth once every ninety minutes. It can also be the second-brightest object in the night sky after the moon. So if you can look up you can watch it move across the sky.

- Every star you see in the night sky is bigger and brighter than our sun, but they are further away than the sun so they do not look as bright.

Sometimes I find keeping secrets is hard. I might have a very exciting project like a big film or TV role, and I would like to let the world know how happy I am. However, the people behind it all, making the film, keep everything secret until the filming is finished and they are working on the edit, because we do not want to spoil it all. It is quite exciting having a secret, but at the same time it is frustrating having to keep it for a year or more. For example, I started filming *Line of Duty* one spring and couldn't tell anyone until the next spring, but it was fair enough keeping that top-secret. I have had to keep my role in *Masters of the Air* secret for about eighteen months.

Inside I might feel a bit fed up about not being able to talk about having an exciting role, but I try not to show it. Usually I say 'I think all my work is top-secret', which feels a bit like being in MI5, but I have just thought of another phrase to say which is 'Who knows?' That seems to make people laugh.

There are some secrets that I might not have told anyone just yet. The main reason for that is because they are for someone else's own benefit. Most of my good friends tease me about keeping secrets, and we do tend to laugh it off, but some friends don't understand and get a bit annoyed. There are some people I do trust to keep secrets, like my mum, but there are others that I do not. So I don't tell them anything about my work. In a way, keeping it separate makes things easier because then I can just be myself with them. That's good because friendship is very important to me.

On that subject, friendship for me means friendship for life. And that basically means going for meals, enjoying trips out and having a laugh with each other, and you can always share your feelings with each other as well. During lockdown we had to stay in touch via Zoom and WhatsApp, which was important to do, and fun too. I like to find out what my friends are up to, and what they are having for lunch and tea. With my friends from Blue Apple I tend to be a calming influence, especially on first nights, when half the cast might be looking forward to going on stage but the other half might be nervous. I think that is part of being professional and being a friend.

Another part of being a friend means helping others when they have difficult times. I want to show that people with Down syndrome and other learning disabilities really are capable of doing this, and how we can support each other in real life.

The loss of a loved one can be very painful. If you are the kind of person who feels really sorry for the loss you can relate to their pain. Then you can console them and help them to mourn their grief as well. One of my friend's mother sadly passed away, and we helped her by listening and also changing the subject when it seemed right. Choosing the right words to say can be tricky, and people need to talk about difficult things. It's a way of making your feelings known and letting it all out, getting it off your chest, but not too much.

I'm interested in what makes people tick. I'd also like to work out what makes people scared or angry. Getting angry means getting stressed out. It happens when you really can't control yourself, and it is one way of letting your emotions out. I want to relate to one of my old friends better when he gets frustrated, and to make people even more aware of what life is like living with those feelings. I have seen him in this situation so many times, and I might have known that side of him the longest. But he also really is a nice person to know. I always help him out in his love life and he helps me out in mine, which is another fun side to him, and we get on very well. Sometimes I think I'm like the laid-back, relaxed side of him, and sometimes he can be the unpredictable side of frustration. I might be like Shearer, whereas my old friend, on the other hand, might be like Roy Keane, to take an example from football.

I truly care for and look out for my old friend. If you hurt his feelings you hurt my feelings as well. If people are horrible to me it hurts his feelings too. We are a bit like Ant and Dec, because we always seem to bring out the fun side in each other.

I feel that people should be able to concentrate on the good things in life, and not to get too focused on all the bad things that are happening in the world right now. One way to stop people being at war with each other is by using choice words, and really thinking about what you are doing to other people. It helps if you can see how they are feeling and coping through life as well.

I think the world needs peacemakers. I actually started being a peacemaker at school. This is my speciality, apparently. I hate other people making dramas out of absolutely nothing at all. I hate that happening with a great passion. One thing that can work is talking to someone calmly and trying not to get too annoyed if their opinion is different to yours. And yet another way is to really listen to someone having a good old rant and getting stuff off their chest about what annoys them.

I can also get quite frustrated and fed up with listening, but I have got a good knack of keeping it inside me. I tend to see the good in people and goodness they bring in life. I would like this book to turn things around and help show this good in people and bring more goodness into the world. I've definitely been helped by some kind people, and each time I have learned something new.

Tommy has introduced us time and again to the kindness of strangers. Not from the people who think they are saying kind things, while pitying you for having a son who has Down syndrome, but from people who have cared and helped in practical ways, like Martin Nobbs going out of his way to find Tommy his first audition; like his first teacher, Mrs Windley at Hillside School, who always talked about what he could do and was as excited as we were each time he learned a new skill; like Mark Rylance believing in him and Lawrie and giving them the fun of taking part in his Pop-up Shakespeare; like Rory Kinnear, who took time to write such an encouraging letter when Tommy played Hamlet; like the person who found him a potato peeler he could use more easily; and like the person, whoever you are, who rescued him when he was lost. I hope you read this book so that I can thank you through this story.

One day just before Christmas a few years ago, we were waiting for Tommy to get home so that we could go to the carol service with him and his grannie. We waited and waited. Eventually I phoned him. He picked up, but could not speak.

At one point that day, for my sins, I was with my good old friend James, who is my partner in crime. We were so busy talking that a mistake was made, and I hopped onto the wrong bus. It literally went entirely the wrong route. I was ten miles away. My mum phoned me but I could not answer. I didn't know what to do or where I was or how to explain. I froze. I could not speak.

I was wondering what on earth to do when his phone rang back. It was the person sitting next to him on the bus, who simply told me that Tommy seemed a bit upset. He had already called his wife to bring their car to drive Tommy home, and where did we live?

I put the phone down with feelings of relief and anxiety running through my head. Who was this man? He must be a safe person to have made all these hugely kind arrangements. I rushed around to find a bottle of wine and wrap it up as a thank you, but when Tommy arrived home

I never even caught site of his rescuer. He waited to see our front door open, then drove off again.

I think I learned how not to get on the wrong bus by getting on the wrong bus. In life you really do have to learn painful things the hard way because then you know from it to not do them again. That could also be one of my many mottos in life, I reckon.

On a different day, I was going to lunch club when the mistake happened. I knew where lunch club was, but I actually walked the opposite way. All the way to the motorway. I kind of realised where I was, and I thought to myself that this might be where the science centre is, not where lunch club is held. I turned round and eventually I reached lunch club. I made it just in time. I might have needed a rest after that.

One Christmas I learned something else the hard way in life, by not knowing that not all buses run on Boxing Day. I decided to go into town to get my TV magazines, so I was waiting at the bus stop for a bus to come by. I waited a long time and a police officer walked up and asked if I was OK. I said I was, so they went away, but when they came back I was still there. They realised I was not OK and brought me home.

Once I called the police when I had been playing football because I didn't know where the person meant to take me home afterwards was. That person might have been a bit cross inside, which is a shame as he was a nice person, but I didn't know what else to do. I had to call someone. The police may not have been the right people to phone.

Another incident happened when my mum went outside and fell over with a bloodcurdling scream. I was upstairs and looked out of my bedroom window. I literally thought she was a goner. It scarred me for life. There was blood everywhere, so I decided to phone my brother to say what happened. I told him I thought she had died. He really did calm me down after that. Poor Will. I found out after a few minutes that it was just a fall. She had tripped on a cable the builders had left out on some steps and fallen down. There was quite a lot of blood, so she had to lie still while my dad tried to stop the bleeding.

*   *   *

Those are some of the scarier things that have happened in my life, but I've definitely learned a few lessons. But there are lots of personal highlights from adventures with my family too! One was learning how to fly a broomstick at Alnwick Castle, which is where Hogwarts School from *Harry Potter* is based. That really was good fun. Another came during a Boys' Day Out with my dad and brother, when we went to New College in Oxford. We had a really nice look around the flowers in the gardens and I discovered that New College Gardens had been used in the fourth Harry Potter film, *The Goblet of Fire*. That might be interesting for the readers of this memoir to find out too, I reckon. I also like going to very old historic houses and doing some research on them before and after with my mum.

Another favourite place of mine is the National Portrait Gallery in London. I like looking at the paintings of people and thinking about how they might be feeling, and their emotions. Then we research the pictures and find out about the different people's lives and whether we think they truly were happy or sad.

Every ten years we go on a holiday adventure. Sometimes we go to the Lake District to walk in the mountains, which is a wicked way to get out in the fresh air. Once when I was very little we were by a stream and I kicked my little wellies in the air. They completely vanished. My brother tried looking for them, but who knows where they went. I really did enjoy wearing them and we had a good laugh about it in the end.

When we went to Namibia (where I had to do my *Line of Duty* audition) we saw some elephants at the waterhole at Etosha, which was also wicked. Learning to make fire and making a poisoned arrow with the Juǀ'hoansi San Bushmen really was good fun, and we saw the largest meteorite in the world, which is called the Hoba meteorite. It weighs 54,000 kilograms and is pretty big really.

We also went to the oldest desert in the world, the Namib desert, where the sand is red because it is so old that iron in the sand has mixed with oxygen in the air, and the older it is the brighter orange or red it is. These are also the tallest sand dunes in the world. We walked through the dunes and to a petrified forest where the trees were so old they had turned completely white. The stars were brilliant because there was no pollution and there were no clouds in the desert. I fell over on the way to the telescope to see the stars, but we did see the Milky Way.

Two more personal highlights from our adventures were being in a jetboat on a river by Middle Earth, where *Lord of the Rings* was filmed, and having some pizza on top of the world's largest active volcano in Hawaii. Wicked.

Interesting facts about deserts:

- The coldest desert on earth is in Antarctica, where it can get to minus 89.2 Celsius. I'm not sure I will be going there.

- The hottest desert in the world is Death Valley in the USA, which I visited once. I went swimming in a hot spring while Will and Dad played tennis. I think they got pretty hot.

Chapter 25

A week in my shoes

When I'm not filming, I have a quiet life at home, hanging out with my friends and family.

Mondays are one of my favourite days of the week. Monday afternoons could be called the Boys' Cooking Day, because me and Dad choose a recipe from Jamie Oliver's *5 Ingredients* to make for our dinner. It was a birthday present from my very own dad and is really useful to have. We take turns to decide what to make from the book, and the clue is exactly what's in the title. There really are only five ingredients we need to make our dinner. But if there's an ingredient that we have not have got, we do tend to go to the supermarket.

Recently I have made Easy Sausage Carbonara, and I had to do quite a lot of chopping to make the meatballs, and stir them around as well. At 6 p.m. we started to eat it. I highly recommend that other people make it too, actually.

Chopping and stirring are the most difficult part. You are learning new fine motor skills as you try your hand at cooking, but your fingers have to get stronger and used to chopping. We've all enjoyed Crispy Skin Lemon Sole, Crazy Simple Fish Pie, Broad Bean Salad and Beef, Beets and Horseradish as well as the carbonara.

I've also made Italian Baked Rice, and it really is worth having. The five ingredients are onions, fennel salami, Arborio risotto rice, mascarpone cheese and Parmesan cheese. A quick tip for people making this recipe is to make sure the saucepan is tipped away from you when you are pouring in the boiling water.

To work up an appetite we also do our exercise regime on Monday mornings, which might include doing some weightlifting, upper-body stretches, leg exercises and sometimes burpees, planks, running on the spot and jumping on the spot for one minute, bicycle kicks, and some press-ups as well.

Whenever I am at home, I also keep fit by going to Low Level Circuits. This started all the way back while I was working in Winchester Library. My mum discovered that I was out of breath walking downhill to the library. She thought that was a bit serious and she decided she needed to do something about it. At that time I might not have had enough sport in my life, so I was getting tired a lot. So, with Winchester and District Mencap, Mum set up low-level circuit training for people with learning disabilities. It's still going twenty years later. We warm up to pop music, then we do weightlifting, rowing on a bench, boxing with a punchbag, bench presses, press-ups, sit-ups and we also have a dance station, which is handy because we all love dancing.

I think dancing is a great thing for you. It makes me feel even more alive and happy, it is good for your bones and makes you fit.

As well as Boys' Cooking Nights, I enjoy our Boys' Nights Out. This is usually Dad, me and Will. It might include going to Piecaramba! to have our supper, where I usually have a Mountie, which is a meat-based pie with mashed potato and mushy peas. A Mountie is quite filling, but you do get to digest it.

And then we go to the Everyman Cinema to watch a movie. Films we've enjoyed include *The Rise of Skywalker*, *Fantastic Beasts and Where to Find Them* and *Thor: Love and Thunder*. Taika Waititi really is an inspiration for me.

When it comes to watching the trailers for upcoming films we have a rating system. Thumbs up means yes, we will watch it. Thumb-shaking means we might not be sure about watching it. Thumbs down: we will not be watching it.

I also research TV news and film news. I like to recommend things to my mum, or to my dad and my brother for Boys' Night Out, although my brother usually gets there first. It is about time I got there ahead of him.

If there's a really big film coming out around Christmas time, the Boys' Night Out might include two generations of brothers – me and Will, and my dad and his brother.

At other times, we might all watch a film together at home. On a special night we will watch Will's latest film. I remember when we went round to my brother's house to watch his documentary, *Investigating Diana: Death in Paris* on Channel 4. Afterwards we asked him about directing it, how they found all the people interviewed and how they filmed everything. It actually is a documentary worth watching or, in other words, to give it a review that counts, it is 'a documentary well worth watching'. It is gripping, fast-moving, powerful and asks big questions about how to get to the truth when so many people couldn't believe what happened and were so upset.

The other thing I'll always be watching, of course, is the football on *Match of the Day* on BBC One. I do enjoy looking forward to the next Premier League game, and a tasty Newcastle match.

Every week I tend to go for a walk to the newsagent to pick up my TV magazines, but sometimes I'll pop into the coffee shop with my dad, and then, for my elevenses, I'll have a sausage roll with crispy pastry.

Once a month, when I am not filming, I work for a charity. I update upcoming events on their social media, which include the Summer Trips Out, their Gateway and Drop In.

I remember one summer, when it was really hot, we filmed our video clips in the grounds of the church, which was wicked although there was some traffic noise. Nobody walked past us. We filmed outside because the post was all to do with sport. Hopefully it helped people to become more involved in taking part. It is one way of keeping fit, and the teamwork is good for your own mental health as well, because you have friends. Friends help and support each other. They are there to commiserate if you lose and if you win they might join in with your happiness.

I also go to the singing group once a week. On the way back I might get my TV magazines from WHSmith's, and then have a really good catch-up with my friend from the group, solving problems from around the world.

Twice a week I'm in college if I'm at home, so on other days I might have lunch with friends. Over lunch we will solve more problems, and catch up with the latest football transfers, the latest goings-on at Blue Apple rehearsals and our love lives as well. And on Sundays, I sometimes carry the cross in church.

One of my other favourite things to do is making my very own lunch and dinner, and not forgetting ordering pizza on a Saturday night. Over the last ten years I have been enjoying flipping pancakes. It has been a flipping good time.

Fridays are a day off, but even when I'm home with my family there's work to do. Almost every day I'm looking at scripts or learning lines for my next part, writing or meeting new people!

It does seem that I'm not getting so many quiet weeks at home any more, though. I think this is a good thing and quite enjoyable. In the space of a few days sometimes I have lots of different things to do. Let me tell you about just one week in autumn 2022.

Tommy, this was quite a week, with four trips to London for work and one to Newcastle, but it was fun flying north on such a lovely day. It seemed even quicker than the train to

London. You also fitted in sessions in college. How did you feel about all this?

Well, it was quite enjoyable. I like being busy.

On Friday I went up to the city of the richest football team in the world, in the form of Newcastle United. I was there to finish off my *Panorama* documentary, but the very first thing that I did was to go on a stadium tour of St James' Park. It was of course wicked. St James' Park is currently the second-biggest stadium in the Premier League. I felt really proud and honoured to be able to visit it. We went up very high above the seats and looked down onto the pitch. The grass was very green. Then we went into a box and saw that everything – tables, chairs, the bar – was in our team colours of black and white.

I actually saw where the new owners sit, as well as where Eddie Howe, the manager, and the substitutes sit during matches.

Then we went to Gateshead for the filming.

On Saturday I finished the last bit of filming with Immy for my *Panorama* documentary. Afterwards Immy and I had lunch to celebrate all our hard work on the film.

Then, on Monday, I went to do some ADR for *Masters of the Air*. For that, I went up to London. ADR stands for automated dialogue replacement and basically means that you go into a studio and have to find different ways to say your lines that will fit the filming. You have repeat it several times and it is all recorded for the final edit of the film.

This time there was a director talking to me on Zoom from Los Angeles, and I just had to redo one word in a scene we shot last year. It was wicked seeing it on a huge screen, and then I had to time the word they wanted to re-record quite quickly.

The director said he liked my scenes in the film. So that was wicked too.

Lots of other actors came to do their lines as well. It was good fun talking about our memories of filming, and how everyone was so friendly.

I thought you did brilliantly and I loved being in that soundproof room. It was pretty cool speaking to the director in California too.

The next day, Tuesday, you were back in London for a consultation on the Down Syndrome Act. What did you say?

It was all about what the lives of people living with Down syndrome really are like, what could make things better and what we want out of life.

You listened to lot of people with Down syndrome talking. What did you find out?

It was interesting looking into what they went through in their lives. One man wanted to change where he lived because it was too far from his friends and family and the activities he wanted to do. He could not afford the taxi fares to see people. I think he should be able to move, because it is not really fair on him.

I don't think people have been listening at all, but they should start to do so right now. What I found most impressive was when people made speeches at the very end of the consultation. They were able to speak out on camera for the first time.

One woman said 'I am so happy because people are listening to me.'

Wednesday – a day off. Thank goodness!

On Thursday I had college. That was fun, and it was good to see my friends there.

On Friday there was more ADR – but for a different project. I was recording a voiceover for my *Panorama* documentary, *Will the NHS Care for Me?*. It was enjoyable and useful as well. It is important to help the viewers to find out even more about what it is like for people with learning disabilities when they need healthcare.

I went into a voiceover booth, which is completely soundproof. I put on some headphones so that the director could talk to me. It was just me in the soundproof room, with the microphone and a TV screen so that I could see the film. I enjoyed watching it because it reminded me of our investigation and all the people I met.

The soundproof room had a glass wall, so I could see the director sitting on a comfy sofa while I was working! But they did give me some grapes, fizzy water and oranges to keep me refreshed.

And at last I was able to let people know about the documentary.

On Saturday we finished the ADR, but there was a train strike so they had to arrange for a car to get us home. I was tracking the football results on the journey. There was so much traffic it took three hours to get home instead of just over one hour.

Next, I had to prepare for a proper meeting with a really top director, so I did my research to see what he had been up to. I found out his full name, his birthday and how old he is, and as much else as I could. I also checked out his IMDb to see which films he might be making next and looked at his interviews online to see what was important to him. I had already watched lots of his movies, but I watched them again, along with even more.

We met in the boardroom of his company's offices. I left feeling wicked and excited about it and looking forward to whatever might come next, but it's all top-secret for now. Then we went off to have lunch at the Wallace Collection, where they have Dutch artists such as Rembrandt, lots of armour, lots of miniature paintings and some gold furniture.

Then after that really busy week I had a new challenge. I was writing a speech for a conference in Manchester with more than four hundred people there.

We had just travelled over 1,200 miles by plane, train and car while working on so many different projects, and the next Monday we took the train to Manchester. I don't feel too good on trains, but we had learned something in the summer to help with the train journey: relax your back and think happy thoughts! Having a good book helps too.

Fact about trains

The world's fastest train as I write is the Shanghai Maglev, which travels on magnets at 286 miles per hour.

We brought a picnic, but we saved it up to last the whole four hours. I was supposed to be filming you preparing your speech for a new documentary, but the angles were very tight as there is not much room between the seats, and I wasn't sure how it would turn out. You were rereading the speech and seemed happy. I knew you would enjoy taking the audience on quite a journey.

It really was wicked making my speech at the Old Trafford Conference Centre for the Community Integrated Care organisation. It turned out we were staying in the Old Trafford hotel, next to the Old Trafford cricket pitch.

We arrived just as it was getting dark and I did what I always do: I went to the window to see what was outside. I was quite amazed by our rooms, each with their own terrace overlooking the cricket pitch, so if there was a match all you had to do was stroll out, into the fresh air and sit at a table to watch.

Next morning we had breakfast, and you had another look at your speech and relaxed a bit before walking over to the conference centre and down a long corridor past all those windows which looked on to the cricket pitch. Then they kept you waiting at the door while they played clips from your showreel. Finally someone made a speech welcoming you. I could just see over your shoulder and there really were more than four hundred people there, sitting at tables, waiting for you. They certainly gave you a dramatic introduction, but I don't think you were nervous. I think you were having a ball the way you twirled and bowed as you arrived on stage.

I am well known for making quite a big entrance when I make my speeches. I actually enjoyed it, but I was looking forward to having lunch afterwards.

Well, you did get your lunch – they were really kind
and packed a cardboard box full of sandwiches and
strawberries for you to eat on the train home. I think there
was also some sort of really sticky chocolate cake!

I began by talking about the football. That was
hilarious. I do tend to make people laugh as well. And
I might have quoted some of my Hamlet lines, which
was wicked.

Here is part of my speech. I hope you will read it and
agree with the important things I said.

I have three themes today: what I think people
need to live their *best lives possible*; people who
helped me; and life as an actor. *So, Friends,
Romans, countrymen, lend me your ears.* [that
made them laugh]

To live their BEST LIVES POSSIBLE, people with
learning disabilities should be treated fairly,
equally and with respect. We're not all the
same, we have our own individual ideas, gifts,
personalities, dreams and ambitions.

BUT we need your help to dig out those gifts and live our lives to the full, have healthy food, keep fit and support our choices. Choices like: where we live – so we can see friends, families and get to work and activities; who we live with – so we get on; and when we eat – so we can get to activities.

If you support us, we need *you to* listen to us, and believe in us.

I went on to tell the audience about my life and the amazing people who have helped me. Then I said:

Don't say you can't. Say *you can* and help us.

Then we *will* be living our best lives possible.

Thank you.

Chapter 26

Intrigued by directing

For one of my latest career moves, in October 2022 I went on a course for emerging directors up in Nottingham that was run by the Regional Theatre Young Directors Scheme with Access All Areas. The main reason I decided to take this course is all to do with giving myself a way of helping Richard Conlon, who is the artistic director of Blue Apple Theatre. I would also like to know how directors' minds work as they put on shows, be behind the camera on set, and understand how the filming works on set.

For the course I worked in Nonsuch Studios Studio 4, and it was a good place to move around in. I stayed in a Premier Inn and they really do have a nice breakfast, which includes sausages, bacon, hash browns and tomatoes, a strawberry yoghurt and a croissant as well as a refreshing drink of orange juice. Not forgetting some coffee to get me energised for the work ahead.

The people on the course were quite a bunch of characters, and interested in life. They wanted to know what Blue Apple was all about, so I told them about Bill Nighy's letter and how we founded the theatre company.

I learned about the different styles of directing, which was intriguing, actually. Like intense, firm but fair, or relaxed and empathetic, which means listening and understanding how the actors are feeling. I also learned about the skills needed in co-directing, which might be useful to know in the future. Those skills include helping out the main director to ease the pressure, which makes it better for the main director and makes the actors feel comfortable as well.

The most interesting thing I learned was how to map out a vision of a show, and then how to go through different stages to make it a reality. We had to think about the location the story is set in, what costumes the actors should wear, the lighting, the characters and casting and the story itself. It was really good fun planning what kind of shows might happen in the future and thinking about all these things.

As part of the course, I had to come up with an idea for a show. I went for a heist movie set in the Caribbean, because I thought it would be great fun to make.

On the Wednesday evening we went to watch *Much Ado About Nothing* in Nottingham. I enjoyed playing Don Pedro with Blue Apple Theatre in this play, but this time I actually watched it from a director's point of view. And that might mean looking at how the actors interact with others on stage, and with the audience as well. At one point in this production, Beatrice was standing in the audience, which was interesting.

The next day, Thursday, we talked about how the show went and how it was staged. We discussed the lighting setup, how the costume and makeup looked, and how the people on stage interacted with the audience, like the actors walking through the audience so that the audience felt involved in the story. I enjoyed that. When all that works out well enough it makes for a really good show to watch.

That evening we went to Happy Dough Lucky, where I had a nice pizza and a lemonade.

And on Friday morning we talked about our very own visions for the future and setting up our own dream shows.

During the course, we improvised a show with no scripts. When you have scripts you are under more pressure to learn lines, and I really would like my shows to be stress-free for my actors. I think working without a script might be easier for some people. You have to improvise and react to other actors, which can be more fun. At times it's a bit pressured, but not too much because you tend to have a laugh whilst reacting to each other, and you can make up your own script with your own words in it. Of course, other people might find this more stressful!

I also want the other actors to be able to find out their strengths and weaknesses, what kind of show they would like to put on for people to watch and enjoy, and which characters they might be best playing. It will be me doing most of the work, but it is also up to the actors to decide what to do with their characters and the emotions behind them. That way we would have an ensemble cast with all of us working collaboratively.

Doing this course made me think about the last Blue Apple production I had been to see, back in the summer. This was a Blue Apple interpretation of *Macbeth*, and it had been really good fun to be a part of. I had played William Shakespeare, but I had pre-recorded this for them as I had been away filming something secret and I could not get to the rehearsals. The play was very funny, making jokes about Covid and Shakespeare-themed plays. Afterwards I went backstage to see the cast and congratulate them on what a brilliant show it was, and on all their hard work. I still feel connected to Blue Apple in some ways. I can't commit to the plays, but I do miss seeing the people. I had a nice catch-up with my friend James, one of the cast members, too. I'm still interested in how their rehearsals are going, and now I've done the directing course I would like to help be an associate director at Blue Apple.

I think *Macbeth* was quite a typical Blue Apple show. Some of the jokes in the show were truly hilarious. My favourite was 'Why did Shakespeare stop outside the bathroom? Because he was deciding whether To Pee Or Not To Pee.' Richard might have made that one up.

I felt really pleased to see how well Blue Apple Theatre are doing and how the actors have been coping with all the rehearsals needed to put on *Macbeth*, but now maybe it's my time to direct.

Chapter 27

Inspired to write

I have always been quite intrigued by famous writers, about what they have written, why they wrote it and who might have inspired them to write.

Now I myself am inspired to write by several writers, including famous playwrights and authors and several people who have written their memoirs and autobiographies.

When I was on BAFTA Elevate, and we felt that there were not enough roles for people like me, they suggested that we might need to start writing them for ourselves. So I did. I met as many people as I could on Zoom and in person to talk about working together and learn about writing. Now I am busy on three writing projects.

Sometimes I have to do some research for this new work. Once part of my research was checking out how policing works. This included watching police dramas, which is fun. I also met a really nice person to chat to. He was a retired police officer. It was quite cold, but not too cold, when we walked down to meet him at the crime and justice department of the university. The place was quite apt for what we were talking about, I thought to myself, as we walked through it.

We sat round a table to talk and I asked him what can go wrong for a police officer. I learned a lot. I think that, when working in the police, you have to expect the unexpected. For example, you should make sure there is not a wall behind you because you might not be able to escape. On the other hand, the wall can be your protection from being attacked from behind. So it could be a safety hazard, but you could also be there for a really good reason.

You have to find an escape route in case you need it. When you knock on a door, you make sure you stand beside it, not in front of it, because who knows who might be behind the door. If they have got one, someone inside might point a gun at the door.

I thought he was an interesting and nice person to speak to.

More recently there was a workshop I did with Sally Phillips and Ronni Ancona and other writers that was really useful for my writing. Sally is a comedy actress known for *Veep* and *Bridget Jones's Diary*, and Ronni is an actress and comedian who does amazing impressions. Sally and Ronni did *Smack the Pony* together.

We started by introducing ourselves and finding out about the work we had been up to. That was quite intriguing. Then we threw some ideas around for the workshop and started working out character and story, and filming them.

Sally and Ronni chipped in with a few extra ideas that we played around with, which were interesting to film as well. The space we were working in was not at all warm. It was freezing, so I kept my coat on.

That was on the first day. On the second day it was a bit warmer, which was helpful, but the heaters were really noisy. On the second day I did get my coat off because it was a bit too hot.

The workshops were enjoyable to do. I had to watch and see how each scene worked out. I tend to think quite a lot and then mention what I think of everything. I enjoy letting things go through my mind a bit first. During my thinking process, if someone asks me what I think before I am ready, I will say 'Not quite yet', because it takes some time to think things over, but I really will say what is on my mind in the end.

The first time I saw the script that was being put together was at breakfast that day. I read it with a writer's eye just to check out what was going through the writer's mind, and then started thinking about it with an actor's mind to find out what the character's feelings are. With a director's mind you have to make sure how the whole piece works.

During the workshops, it would have helped if I could have done some of the acting. On the other hand, I enjoyed being behind the camera and letting other people show what they are capable of in front of it.

I did mention some stuff on the writing, which was useful, and had some other suggestions for the production team. Sally did say that it was really helpful having us all there for them to work with.

The first time I worked with Sally Phillips was in November 2017 at a scratch comedy night at the Orange Tree Theatre in Richmond. That was another highlight in my career. We had to rewrite and shorten our script at the last minute, but it worked out well actually and the audience seemed to like it. As I said, I literally feel Sally Phillips is like a godmother to my career.

In 2018 I went to Stockholm with Sally for a comedy festival to talk about a project we want to make together. The plane was late, so when I arrived I had to go straight on stage to introduce myself and give a hello message to Stockholm, which was a bit sudden as I was not expecting this. Arriving at events late can be difficult.

Later I met Jennifer Saunders and her daughter Beattie Edmondson, which was fun, and we all went out to dinner and had Swedish meatballs and lots of laughing together.

The weather in Stockholm was even more freezing than in England. The next day, I ended up going to the Abba Museum and dancing and singing to their videos. My favourite Abba songs to sing to definitely have to be 'Mamma Mia' and 'Dancing Queen', which always get me and my mum dancing.

I would like to write roles for people with Down syndrome where their characters are living their lives to the full, have relationships, romance, adventures, and can speak up about what they want to do in life. As a writer you have to show truth, and I want to show the real truth about people with Down syndrome. Working with Will and writing this book have given me confidence and inspired me to become a writer. It has been enjoyable and I've learned that writing is fun. People have believed in me, and I would like to be an inspiration to other people who wish to be writers themselves.

Chapter 28

What comes next?

As much as I agree that my work should be top-secret before it goes on air, I really would like to let people know the exciting things I am doing next. It would be nice to share the fun with them, and I think they might be quite pleased to know. But some people might not understand about keeping it top-secret, so I can't tell them everything. I'm pleased to have got that off my chest.

So, what can I say about my plans? Well, I really enjoy seeing what might be coming up next in my career. I am excited about discovering who I could be working with, and researching and meeting many casting directors and producers and also up-and-coming writers. My dream is to star in a feature film in the cinema. To play James Bond, be a superhero or fall in love in a romcom. My ultimate dream is to be in a Hollywood movie. I hope that this will be what comes next, maybe along with presenting more documentaries or more journalism. Sometimes you might have to try to make these dreams happen yourself. So that is what I am doing. I'm trying to make something happen, which is wicked and exciting.

I'm making a new documentary with my brother Will for the BBC. It is about me chasing my new acting dream. We are setting out to create and pitch an original idea for a new Hollywood movie inspired by my life story.

It has always been a major dream to work with Will and make the type of a film that I would like to be in. Recently, we filmed some choreography I was doing with Daniel Vais, which is always a highlight, and we were throwing some ideas around for our movie. I'm looking forward to doing more of this. Next time we will do more choreography and look at costumes, which should be fun. We might work out some movement for my character, who is still top-secret by the way. The only thing I can reveal is that he is named Roger, in honour of my teddy bear. Roger might be a sci-fi fantasy character like Sherlock Holmes, or someone in disguise as a secret agent like James Bond. I would like to play something with mystery and stillness, and a bit of comedy as well. Someone who makes his presence felt and saves the day.

Will does not do things by half, and he can be really focused on getting the right shots. He enjoys filming beautiful places and things like the autumn trees. Filming the trees is a typical Will filming event, which I know all too well! I like working with him in the sunlight under the trees, but he always says 'one last time'. I do have to laugh at that, as I would like to know whether it truly is one last time or not. I really do have to look at the funny side of it.

Will has also given me my very own camera now, so sometimes I am the one filming him, or filming what is going on. I am really enjoying being behind the camera for a change, learning how to make a documentary as well as be in it. We have been filming with some brilliant people, like the actors Will Sharpe and Kit Harington and a writer called Amanda

Graham. As I am writing this, we are just about to jump on a plane to Hollywood to pitch our idea! That feels quite wicked and exhilarating. I am really looking forward to this.

Me and Will laugh a lot while working together. He understands me and we are having fun creating the story for a movie together. We're trying to make our dreams happen ourselves.

Well, who knows what will happen next! Whatever it is, I hope it will be exciting, I hope Will and I get our film made, and whatever happens I hope you have all enjoyed reading my story so far. Remember we are all different, we all have gifts, we might just need help digging them out.

Maybe I could finish off with two of my mottos in life:

Actions speak louder than words.

Don't judge a book by its cover. (Except this one, as I said earlier!)

What else am I hoping for in the future...? Good question.

(Not) The End...

Sayings of Tommy

I have to give you these first three one last time!

- Actions speak louder than words, and I've always lived by that and I always will do.

- Don't judge a book by its cover.

- Everyone has a gift inside them. We just need to help them dig it out.

- Labels separate people.

- Friends are forever.

- Bad things can be good things:
  o If it was going to be a really bad day, he'd swallowed a big frog.

o   If it was going to be just a bit bad, then he'd swallowed a smaller frog.

- Good things come to those who wait.

- Communication is the key to success.

- Howay the lads!

- Save the best till last...

- TO BE!!!

PS Final intriguing fact

The tallest mountain in the world is not Mount Everest, it is Mauna Kea in Hawaii because it starts underwater! Mount Everest is the highest.

Acknowledgements

I hope you enjoyed reading my book. That's my life so far. It has been fun and intriguing writing it. Thank you to my family and my friends, and to all the people who have supported me in my life and in my career including all my brilliant teachers, and the producers, writers, directors and commissioners who have believed in me and given me the chance to play some brilliant roles in film, television and on stage. Julie Anne Robinson, Mark Haddon, Roanna Benn, Neil Dudgeon, Julia Ford, Jed Mercurio, Ken Horn, Mark Rylance, Cary Fukenaga, Bugsy Riverbank Steele, Guy Bolton, Daniel Vais, Ben Reid, Tibault Travers, Natalie Kennedy, Christopher Faith, Mariayah Kaderbhai and all at BAFTA, you really have helped change our world. Thanks to Vicky McClure, Kelly Macdonald, Nicholas Hoult, Perry Fitzpatrick, Gregory Piper, Bethany Asher, Laurence Spellman, Sally Phillips, Simon Kunz, Robbie O'Neill, Delroy Atkinson, Otto Baxter, Sam Barnard, Rishard Beckett, Warwick Davis, Hugo Speer, Austin Butler, Callum Turner and all the other actors who were kind and wicked to work with. Thank you to the factual commissioners and production teams at the BBC, BBC Studios, Maverick TV, Dartmouth Films, Panorama and Hardcash for giving me the chance to make some important documentaries. Thanks to the Royal Ballet and Royal Opera House for a brilliant experience learning ballet with you and performing *The Rite of Spring* with other dancers from Culture Device. Thanks to the Globe Theatre in London for allowing us to perform for our Blue Apple tenth birthday celebration on stage in the Sam Wanamaker Playhouse. And to Bill Nighy, for inspiring us to found Blue Apple Theatre.

Very special thanks to my mother who made my life worth living, and to my brother, Will, for always being fun to work with, having a laugh and creating so many wicked projects for stage, television and now, we hope, film, taking me to the International

Emmy Awards and also supporting the same football team from the very beginning. More very special thanks and love to my dad, Cara, Soraya, Ben, Molly, Jules and Janet, Sally S, Meriel, Martin Nobbs, Margie and John, John and Angela, and Grannie and Grandpa for your support and for always believing in me and being happy for me. Thank you to Ken and Rachael Ross, Fionn and Jonathan Crombie Angus, Dr Liz Corcoran, Dr Liam Fox MP, Florence Garrett, Heidi Crowter, James Carter, Max Ross and everyone at the National Down Syndrome Policy and Advisory Groups. It's been really good and important campaigning with you.

I'd also like to thank so many other talented people with Down syndrome who inspire me: Sarah Gordy, George Webster, James Martin, Ellie Goldstein, Zack Gottsagen, Liam Bairstow, Leon Harrop, Joe Sproulle, Sara Pickard, the artists of Drag Syndrome, everyone at Culture Device and Radical Beauty, and so many more of you.

Thank you to all my friends and collaborators at Blue Apple Theatre, especially James B, James E, Katy, Lawrie, Ros, Anna. It's been wicked. Thank you to all the directors at Blue Apple Theatre, Barbara Garfath,

Keren Ben Dor, Philip Glassboro, Anita Rogers, John Tellett, Peter Clerke and Richard Conlon for your care and passion in creating brilliant roles for us all, Chris Pearce, Sarah Criddall, Betty Chadwick, Emma Snagge and everyone at Winchester GoLD, and everyone at national Mencap. Thank you to all the kind people at church where I carry the cross and have read the lesson.

Thank you to my book agent, Kate, and everyone at Headline and Wildfire, especially Alex, Flora, Areen, Patrick, Vicky and Joe for giving me the opportunity to tell my story. Thank you to my acting agents, Nicki, Rachael, Clarissa and Lotti.

There have been many highs which we have celebrated together, and lows which we have suffered together as well.

Friends are forever.

Tommy has worked with the following organisations:

BAFTA Elevate

BAFTA Elevate is a bespoke programme that aims to help support individuals from under-represented backgrounds, to reach the next stage of their career. In 2019, BAFTA Elevate focused on a select group of actors from under-represented groups seeking to progress in high-end television drama, comedy and features. Tommy Jessop was selected along with 20 other actors as someone who had proved that they possess extraordinary talent in the craft of acting.

Tommy's debut in the BAFTA-nominated primetime drama *Coming Down the Mountain* (BBC) alongside Nicholas Hoult was astonishing, and he's gone on to make a mark in everything he's done for stage and screen since. Actors from underrepresented groups can face far more barriers in pursuing a career in acting – where roles are many but only a few are selected.

Tommy has proved that he can turn his hand to any genre and play the lead.

Blue Apple Theatre

Blue Apple Theatre was founded by Jane with Tommy in 2005 because many people with learning disabilities said they were isolated and lonely with no opportunity to take part in the performing arts.

Right from the beginning, the aim was to be ambitious, lift the ceiling of expectation and change the way the public see people with any form of learning disability.

Blue Apple is now recognised as one of the foremost theatre companies in the UK for people with a learning disability, performing and touring drama, dance, film and song locally, nationally and even internationally with partners in the Czech Republic, Poland and Italy.

Theatre can change lives by providing empowering, enriching opportunities, with a sense of purpose and belonging, where friendships are forged and people discover their skills and grow in confidence.

To support Blue Apple please donate here: www.blueappletheatre.com/donate

Mencap

Tommy is a Myth Buster Ambassador for Mencap – the UK's leading charity supporting people with a learning disability. There are 1.5million people in the UK with a learning disability and Mencap works to support them, their families and carers by fighting to change law, improve services, and access to education, employment and leisure facilities.

Mencap's vision is for the UK to be the best place in the world for people with a learning disability to live happy and healthy lives. Tommy has done so much to help this vision by using his role as a Mencap Myth Buster Ambassador to challenge misconceptions about living with a learning disability

If you have been inspired by Tommy's story and want to support Mencap's work you can donate here www.mencap.org.uk/tommy

National Down Syndrome Policy Group

The National Down Syndrome Policy Group (NDSPG) believe people with Down syndrome should be at the very heart of policy making and is a collaboration of people with Down syndrome with representatives and professionals from some of the UK's leading support organisations. The NDSPG is endorsed by over 125 Down syndrome and learning disability organisations across the UK, as well as key experts. They support people with Down syndrome to have their say at a regional and national level, working in partnership with a large Advisory Group consisting solely of people with Down syndrome who act as self-advocates and ambassadors for the group, and who actively contribute to their joint agenda.

The NDSPG successfully lobbied for the Down Syndrome Act 2022 and was heavily involved in its creation. They continue to work with individuals, organisations, government and professionals to support the formation of the Down Syndrome Act Guidance, and to improve services, policy and legislation.

The NDSPG also provides the secretariat to the All-Party Parliamentary Group on Down Syndrome. www.ndspg.org

Portsmouth Down Syndrome Association

Portsmouth Down Syndrome Association (Portsmouth DSA) is an award-winning charity with royal approval, improving lives, opportunities and outcomes by providing some of the UK's best and most comprehensive specialist services from the point of diagnosis, and training thousands of parents and professionals each year.

Portsmouth DSA works hard to raise awareness, champion inclusion & celebrate diversity because when people with Down syndrome are given opportunities to participate & be fully included, the whole community benefits.

The charity also actively campaigns to improve services and legislation for people with Down syndrome. It has played an integral part in the formation of the Down Syndrome Act 2022 and continues to work closely with the National Down Syndrome Policy Group and government to support the development of the Down Syndrome Act Guidance. www.portsmouthdsa.org

If you would like to donate to Portsmouth DSA, please visit: Portsmouth Down Syndrome Association – JustGiving

Winchester Go LD

Winchester Go LD is a small local charity, enabling adults with learning disabilities to live their lives to the full, with the independence and choices that they want. We promote wellbeing, self-development, friendship, self-confidence, creativity and learning. We have a range of weekly and monthly activities and we provide advocacy, information, safeguarding and skills workshops. (https://winchestergold.org.uk/).

Tommy is a very popular and longstanding member of Winchester Go LD. He brings with him a huge amount of fun, energy and enthusiasm. Tommy has contributed to Winchester Go LD in many positive ways. Amongst other things, he and his mother set up our weekly low level circuits session at our local leisure centre over 20 years ago. These sessions have gone from strength to strength providing much needed physical exercise and social engagement to adults with learning disabilities in our community; with over 25 Winchester Go LD members taking part each week, circuits has become our most popular weekly activity. Tommy has also worked in our office helping us with our social media posts and our regular newsletters. We love having him as part of our team.

Scan below for more information

and access to a downloadable PDF

of our Easy Read edition